Cosmetic Surgery:

The Consumer's Complete Easy Guide From Before to After

By

Cynthia E. Sutton & Wanda S. Lyon

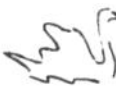

DISCLAIMER

This book was written to provide general information regarding cosmetic surgery, skin maintenance, anesthesia, etc. It is neither intended nor implied to be a substitute for proper professional medical care and under no circumstances should be considered to supercede the information provided to a patient by a certified medical professional.

UNDER NO CIRCUMSTANCES SHOULD READERS ATTEMPT TO PERFORM ANY OF THESE PROCEDURES OR ADMINISTER ANY PRODUCTS MENTIONED HEREIN WITHOUT BEING UNDER THE CARE OF A QUALIFIED, LICENSED MEDICAL PROFESSIONAL.

We, as authors, neither recommend nor disagree with cosmetic surgery. The intent of this text is to inform the consumer so that sound, educated decisions can be made in an informed manner.

This book is as thorough and correct as we could make it. However, there may be errors, both typographical and in content. The information contained herein should **only be used as a guide. Scientific and/or medical data brought forth after publication date may supercede information provided within these pages.**

The authors and Publisher will assume no liability or responsibility, neither legally nor morally, to any person or entity for any loss or damage caused, or alleged to be caused, either directly or indirectly, by the information contained in this book.

THIS BOOK MAY BE RETURNED TO THE PUBLISHER FOR A FULL REFUND SHOULD YOU NOT AGREE TO THE ABOVE CONDITIONS.

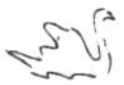

ACKNOWLEDGMENT

Our sincere appreciation to two of the most prominent and respected physicians in the field of plastic surgery: Drs. John G. Penn and John R. Royer. The time that each spent away from his busy Central Florida practice to assist us in providing our readers with state-of-the-art information on cosmetic surgery is a direct reflection of the dedication that each has for his profession. These men embody all that is right with this branch of medicine -a committment to excellence and a sincere concern for the patient.

Many thanks to Dr. William Purkey for his time and input in helping to inform our readers about anesthesia. Although they seldom receive the glory or recognition for a successful surgery, the physician anesthesiologist is a valuable and crucial part of the team at your side in the operating room.

Our appreciation to Dr. J. Barry Boyd, Mr. Paul Licata, and Victoria Snyder for the time and effort spent editing our work.

And, finally, to our families - for their love, support and for the belief that we could achieve our dream.

For Amanda and Natalie,

For whom

all things are possible.

TABLE OF CONTENTS

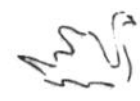

CHAPTER ONE

BEFORE YOU SEE THE DOCTOR

Janice was ecstatic - at the age of forty-nine she was finally in a financial position to do with her appearance something that she had dreamed of since her teen years: she was having plastic surgery on her nose! While she had always felt good about her features in general, she had never been fond of her nose - it seemed over-large for her face, and it had a prominent bump when viewed in profile. A recent career advancement held the promise of a sizeable financial reward, and she had decided to give herself a "new nose" for all those years of hard work in her job. Since her new career responsibilities would place her in a highly visible position, she felt that her new profile would do nothing but assist her in developing the confidence that she would need in speaking to large groups of business associates. Her husband was fully supportive, making her even more relaxed about her decision to undergo cosmetic surgery.

Janice was methodical in her search for a qualified plastic surgeon. She contacted her family physician for the names of surgeons that he would recommend, and she contacted the local hospital for a listing of affiliated doctors who performed cosmetic surgery on the nose. She narrowed her list to two surgeons and made consultation appointments with each. Both of the sessions went well, so Janice scheduled her surgery with the doctor who made her feel the most comfortable during the consultation process.

Today, Janice is extremely positive and enthusiastic when asked about her experience with plastic surgery. She loves her "new nose", and readily attests to the good things that cosmetic surgery did for her self-image.

At the age of twenty-six, Krista felt as though she had reached a dead-end in her career and love life. Although she had worked for her current employer for seven years, she was unhappy in her job but saw no means by which she could change her career path. Krista would readily admit that she was involved in an unfulfilling relationship with her boyfriend. She complained to family and friends about his frequent habit of staring at other women. Krista had convinced herself that her small breasts were the reason for her boyfriend's wandering eyes. She felt inadequate in comparison to women with a fuller bustline, and her feelings of inadequacy contributed to her outbursts of jealousy and rage at her mate. When Krista learned through a mutual acquaintance

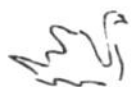

that her boyfriend had recently had an affair with a woman at his office, she resolved to change herself into a person that her boyfriend could not live without. Taking stock of her savings account, she grabbed the phonebook, flipped the yellow pages to "Plastic Surgeons", and began calling. She asked two questions of each receptionist: "Does this doctor do breast enlargements?" and "How much does he charge?"

Krista made an appointment for a consultation with the first surgeon who's fees for breast augmentation matched the balance in her savings account. In the consultation, Krista heard little of what the doctor had to say. Her primary concern was the expense of the procedure and how quickly the surgery could be scheduled.

Krista had her breasts enlarged with silicone implants; the surgery was a complete success from a medical point of view. Krista, however, was seriously disappointed in her results. Her breasts were considerably larger that what she had envisioned. To her regret, her new breasts seemed to have no effect on any of her problems - she still hated her job, and her wayward boyfriend moved out of the apartment that they had shared and married another woman within a few months. With her savings account depleted and breasts that she was no more satisfied with than those she had before surgery, she was as unhappy as ever.

The medical community has seen a rapid upswing in recent years in the number of patients electing to have cosmetic or "aesthetic" surgery (both terms mean the same thing -a procedure undertaken to improve appearance). This should come as no surprise to anyone that owns a television set, reads magazines or visits a health gym. Americans place a high premium on an attractive appearance; some psychological studies indicate that, even subconsciously, we react in a more positive manner to persons who are physically appealing. Not that we should be *too* hard on ourselves for this beauty-fixation: we've all seen pictures in magazines of members of remote African tribes that "disfigure" (to our western tastes) themselves in order to achieve a level of personal attractiveness which is desirable in their society. It was common in some Asian cultures to bind the feet of females in order to create a physical deformity that was considered attractive and desireable. And what about the millions of dollars spent each year on cosmetics in the United States alone? All this in an effort to be more satisfied with our physical appearance.

Each period of human history and each culture has had a standard by which beauty is judged. It is very human, then, to strive to conform to those standards that we have set for ourselves. If not with the features handed to us by nature, then with the help of science.

The field of plastic surgery includes two distinct types of procedures: *reconstructive* surgery, which is used to repair function and appearance of tissue affected by disease, accident or birth defect, and *aesthetic* or *cosmetic* surgery, which

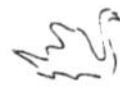

describes those procedures undertaken strictly for an improvement in appearance. Plastic surgery itself has come a long way since its beginnings in the years following World War I, when it was primarily used to reconstruct the bodies of soldiers ravaged by war injuries. The use of surgery solely to enhance appearance really didn't catch on until fairly recently, relatively speaking, and has been gaining in popularity at an astounding rate with each passing decade.

In 1990, 87% of cosmetic procedures were performed on women; 13% on men. The top five most popular procedures for that year were:

1. Liposuction

2. Breast Augmentation (Enlargement)

3. Collagen Injections

4. Eyelid Surgery

5. Nose Reshaping

Based on procedures performed in 1990 by members of the American Society of Plastic and Reconstuctive Surgeons

Electing to have plastic surgery for cosmetic reasons is no longer confined to fashion models, actresses and the wealthy - most surgeons we spoke with feel that at least half of all patients electing to undergo plastic surgery have a household annual income that could be considered average. Since most plastic surgery procedures undertaken for purely aesthetic reasons (to look good) are not covered by insurance, it is obvious that a great many people are willing to make a financial sacrifice to achieve the sometimes dramatic results that plastic surgery can bring about.

In 1990 alone, over a half-million Americans chose to alter their appearance by means of plastic surgery. If you were to ask each one of these patients why he or she chose to undergo a surgical procedure to correct, enhance, diminish or eradicate a self-perceived imperfection, you would most likely receive over a half-million different responses. With the increasingly tight job market, it's not surprising that many prospective plastic surgery patients are looking for ways to remain competitive on the career path. Our youth-oriented society sometimes places a great deal of strain on those approaching middle-age, and some men and women feel compelled to maintain a youthful appearance for the good of their careers.

Your age will likely play a large part in the type of cosmetic surgery that you are considering. Patients in or near the adolescent years (teens through twenties) are more likely to lean toward the correction of a facial feature, such as having a nose reshaped. Patients in their fourties and older are more likely to want a procedure that will help eradicate some of the signs of aging, such as a facelift or chemical peel. The following chart reflects statistics gathered by the ASPRS from

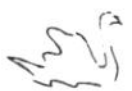

its members on the average age of patients electing the most common cosmetic surgery procedures for aesthetic reasons:

Percentage of Procedures by Age Group

AGE	Facelift	Nose	Eyelids	Breast Augment	Breast Reduction	Chemical Peel
Under19	0%	11%	0%	1%	6%	1%
19-34	1%	57%	5%	65%	46%	4%
35-50	27%	27%	44%	32%	34%	28%
51-64	59%	4%	42%	3%	11%	57%
65+	13%	1%	10%	0%	3%	11%

Statistics furnished by members of the American Society of Plastic and Reconstructive Surgeons.

Your reason for considering plastic surgery is uniquely your own. Perhaps you would like to better fill out your bathing suit as you cruise the Caribbean next summer, or maybe you can no longer bear looking into the mirror and seeing Uncle Bernard's nose smack in the middle of *your* face. You've made up your mind to finally do something about this part of yourself that haunts your self-image.

"Wait a second", you say. "How in the world am I going to explain my new bustline to my mother?" "What will my friends think?" And, "How will Uncle Bernard feel about me having *his nose* pared down to something I'm more comfortable with?" The best possible method of assuring yourself and concerned others that you have made a wise choice is to arm yourself with the information that you need to make a responsible, well-informed decision. Secondly, to make certain that your expectations of the results of your surgery are realistic and positive to your self-image.

Our goal in this book is to give you the information that you need to make a well-informed decision regarding cosmetic procedures. With data gathered from experts in the field of plastic surgery, extensive research, statistical data and illustrations, we will provide you with a thorough and impartial overview of the most common elective plastic surgery procedures undertaken for cosmetic reasons.

Are you a good candidate for plastic surgery? There are several factors that will influence the answer to that question. Your doctor, once you select one, will advise you as to whether you are a good candidate for the specific procedure that you're considering. There are, however, some questions you need to ask of yourself *before* your visit to the surgeon of your choice.

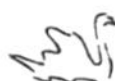

WHY DO I WANT PLASTIC SURGERY?

If your response to this question has anything to do with solving all of your problems, winning the lottery or bringing about world peace, you will be sadly disappointed. Plastic surgery, no matter how successful, will *not* do any of these things for you. What a good surgeon *can* do is assist you in improving your appearance. If you want a new life, you will be better off to see your psychotherapist; if you want a new nose, see your plastic surgeon. Most ethical plastic surgeons will turn away a prospective patient if that person appears to be a psychological risk. One of the more pleasant outcomes of plastic surgery can be improved self-esteem and self-confidence because of a more positive self-image, but changing any other negative aspects of your life is up to you. Those people who do experience a change in certain aspects of their personality after a cosmetic procedure are generally people who were experiencing difficulty in self-esteem or self-confidence due to a feeling of inadequacy about their appearance. For example, if you are shy and introverted because you are afraid that people are staring at your nose (or ears, or whatever), having that feature altered with surgery may give you the self-confidence to reach out to others more often. Just try to make certain that you are considering a change in your appearance to please ***yourself***. It's very tempting at times to think that if we just had nicer breasts, a perky nose or full lips that the person of our dreams would ride in on a white horse and sweep us off of our feet. Unfortunately, that's just not apt to happen. Remember -beautiful people have problems, too. Make the decision to do something positive for yourself and you'll most likely be happier with your results.

Be sure that you are comfortable with the idea of "fooling around with Mother Nature". Are you going to feel guilty about using surgery to change your appearance? If so, do some deep soul-searching before you make your decision. It may help to talk things out with a good friend. Sometimes just saying things "out loud" will help to put a situation in perspective.

ARE MY EXPECTATIONS REALISTIC?

Your goal from plastic surgery should be to improve on the features that you already have. It isn't fair to your surgeon or yourself to expect perfection. There are many variables that will play a part in the degree of success that can be achieved in any operation: your age, general health, skin texture, skin elasticity, bone structure and your attention to post-operative instructions, to name but a few. Results will vary from patient to patient on the same procedure performed by the same surgeon, and *each* patient will interpret the success of his or her surgery differently. If you are thinking of taking advantage of plastic surgery in order to make yourself look like someone else, forget it. Bone structure, skin tone and basic

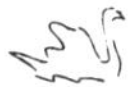

It is very important to check your surgeon's qualifications. Is he/she Board Certified, and by what board? Is this board recognized by the American Medical Association? Is this physician listed in Marquis' Directory of Medical Specialists? (Check your library). Be very thorough in your selection process - it is up to you to protect yourself from unethical or underqualified persons performing cosmetic procedures. Again, ***please take the time to verify board certification, and to assure that the certifying board is recognized by the American Board of Medical Specialties!!***

QUESTIONS FOR THE DOCTOR

You're almost ready for your consultation! After narrowing your list of prospective doctors to three or four, you may want to schedule a consultation appointment with the two cosmetic surgeons who best fit your criteria (qualifications, specialty, etc.). While a surgeon *does* generally charge a small fee for consultation (see the next chapter for more detail on the consultation process) you will get a much better idea of what to expect if you see more than one doctor for this initial step in your surgery process. Some surgeons will offer a second follow-up consultation at no charge, should you wish to revisit either doctor before making your final decision. If you are 100% comfortable with the first doctor you consult with, you can always cancel the consultation appointment with your second doctor. Before you walk into the doctor's office, though, you need to make sure that you are as well prepared for the appointment as you want the surgeon to be. In order to assure that all of the questions that you have regarding your surgery get answered, make a list! You'll probably be much more at ease and feel more confident after this first visit with the surgeon if you have gotten good feedback on your questions. We list some of the more common questions that patients ask in consultation, but we encourage you to add your own as needed:

- Are you board certified, and by what board?
- How experienced are you with this type of procedure?
- In what medical specialty are you certified?
- Am I a good candidate physically for this surgery?
- How much improvement can I expect from this operation?
- Are my expectations realistic?
- May I see pictures of other patients who have undergone this type of procedure?
- How can I get a good idea of the results of my surgery?
- Where will the surgery be performed?
- What type(s) of anesthesia will be used?
- Who will be administering the anesthesia, and what are their qualifications?

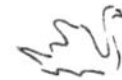

- What risks or complications are common to this surgery, and how often do they occur?
- What type of emergency care is available should it be needed?
- Is there a great deal of discomfort both during and after this procedure?
- Where and by whom will I receive post-operative care?
- How long is the recovery period, and how long will I be out of work?
- Will there be noticeable scars from the surgery? Where will they be?
- What can I expect in the first few weeks following surgery?
- How soon can I resume normal activity?
- Are the results to this procedure permanent? If not, how long do they last?
- How much do you charge for this surgery?
- Are there additional charges, such as for anesthesia?
- If I need follow up care, either as a result of complications or corrective treatment, is there a charge? How much?
- Will insurance cover any part of the cost of this procedure?

A good surgeon will not be offended by your questions - he or she will welcome your concern, since this will help assure that you are an informed patient, and are prepared to weigh the risks against the benefits of cosmetic surgery. Most surgeons much prefer to work with a patient who is well-informed and recognizes the limitations of any procedure, as well as one who has realistic expectations. Again, these are suggestions for your question list. Make sure to jot down anything that you want to cover in the first consultation, and be sure to read Chapter 2 so that you know what to expect with your first meeting with the doctor and his staff.

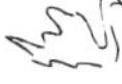

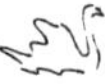

CHAPTER TWO

THE CONSULTATION

> *"Where does beauty begin and where does it end? Where it ends is where the artist begins."*

John Cage
"Lecture on Nothing" Silence (1961)

You've completed your search for the plastic surgeon that you want to perform your cosmetic procedure and it's time for your first visit to his/her office. After all of your painstaking research to find the best doctor for your needs and the hours spent verifying credentials, you're really going to get to sit down and talk to this person! So why are you feeling so apprehensive and embarrassed about the whole thing and actually having doubts about your decision to have the procedure in the first place? Because it's perfectly normal, that's why. Your fantasy about that new nose, slimmer hips, more youthful face or pleasing breasts is about to be put to the harsh light of reality. "Am I being silly and vain to even consider the procedure?" you wonder. Or worse yet, "What if the doctor takes one look at me and wants to schedule me for surgery from head to toe?" *Relax* - your fears and apprehension are to be expected. If you've done your homework and scheduled your consultation with a qualified, ethical doctor with the appropriate amount of experience, your fears are going to be short-lived.

Usually, an initial consultation will take anywhere from fifteen minutes to an hour. Each doctor will have his own routine for the consultation process, but there is a fairly basic format that most plastic surgeons will follow in some order:

1. You will generally see the nurse or some other member of the surgeon's staff first. You'll be asked to complete a medical history listing any known medical conditions or allergies, medications or other substances you're currently taking, whether or not you smoke, if you have a history of unusual bleeding or heavy scarring, if you bruise easily and if you have had any

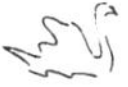

sides to aging is the loss of skin elasticity. For this reason, some patients that schedule a procedure such as a facelift may enjoy a more successful result if the surgery is done when skin elasticity is still at a more youthful level. Even in procedures such as liposuction (fat suctioning) the degree of skin elasticity will be a factor in achieving a pleasing result, since the skin must have the ability to adapt well to the new contour of the body. That is *not* to say that you will not be a good candidate for the procedure if your skin elasticity isn't at its best - but the doctor will most likely let you know that your results could be somewhat less than you may have hoped.

Another important criteria to your procedure may be **bone structure**. Especially in facial procedures, the basic contour of your features will greatly influence the outcome of your procedure. In cases where the patient is particularly interested in altering features which are ethnic in origin, the surgeon will probably exercise a certain amount of conservative restraint. The doctor will evaluate the level of achievable success given the bone structure of your face.

Depending on the type of procedure that you are considering, **body weight** could be a factor in your surgery. Especially for patients thinking of such procedures as **liposuction or breast reduction**, *plastic surgery is not a substitute for a healthy diet and regular exercise.* Nor are they meant to alter the shape of an entire body - liposuction, especially, is intended to be used to remove localized fat deposits which create a distortion in the contour of the body, such as the fatty deposits on some women's hips known as "saddlebags". If a patient is truly obese, the doctor will probably want to see some reduction in body weight before scheduling surgery.

Skin texture and coloring will also be factors in determining your candidacy for a procedure. As a rule, dark skinned people tend to scar more noticeably than persons with a lighter complexion. Also, dark skin may be "heavier", and thus be more resistant to the draping and lifting procedures. Not that life is all bad to those with a darker complexion -usually the lighter the skin, the more early in life the signs of aging appear. The good news for those with fair skin, though, is that the texture of fair skin is generally more favorable for the lifting procedures and chemical peels that can help erase those tell-tale wrinkles and fine lines.

These are generalities, of course, and should in no way either encourage or discourage you in regards to a certain procedure. Each individual must be evaluated with his or her own unique characteristics before the feasibility or success of a specific procedure can be put into perspective. And, of course, there are an infinite number of combinations of skin texture and color, body weight, skin elasticity and bone structure. You and your surgeon must determine if the results that are possible, given your unique set of circumstances, are agreeable enough to proceed with scheduling the surgery.

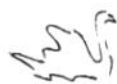

EDUCATION

After you and your plastic surgeon have established communication and the evaluation process has been completed, it's time for your education to commence. The first thing you're probably going to want to learn is "How will I look?". Now that your doctor has completed your physical evaluation, he or she can give you an informed answer. The method that your doctor chooses to utilize in giving you a good estimation of the results of your procedure may be different than the means used by another surgeon. Some will take a pen and paper and diagram out for you what they intend to do during surgery, and a close approximation of the results that they think you'll end up with. Many physicians will use books and/or slides for the same purpose. Other surgeons may use a relatively new tool in projecting surgical results - *computer imaging*.

Using a computer to give plastic surgery patients a "preview" of their new nose, more youthful face or larger/smaller breasts is a fairly recent development. Special video equipment and software (the program that tells the computer what to do) are used to project the patient's image on a screen. The doctor can use various computer tools to "draw in" the new nose or whatever, giving the patient an opportunity to visualize the intended results. Remember that **plastic surgery is a marriage of art and science.** Not even the best plastic surgeon can guarantee that the results of your procedure will exactly reflect what you see on paper or on a video screen. All of the factors that went in to your physical evaluation will play a part in determining your results, as will the way that your body scars, swells and heals. For this reason, some plastic surgeons decline to use computer imaging in patient consultations - they feel that the patient can leave the office with unrealistic expectations for the results of their procedure. If your plastic surgeon does use computer imaging, be aware that, as with all things pertaining to the human body, cosmetic surgery is not an exact science.

RISKS AND COMPLICATIONS

No consultation is complete unless the doctor has a serious discussion with you in regard to the possible risks inherent to your surgery, and the possible unforeseen complications that can result from your procedure. While most patients who are in relatively good health will probably have a statistically small level of risk involved with their surgery, **you must make yourself aware of the possible complications and make your decision to commence with the procedure only after you are fully aware of these circumstances.**

Each type of cosmetic surgery has a unique set of possible complications. The most common of these will be discussed in the chapter of this book devoted to that particular procedure. In addition, anesthesia carries with it inherent risks to the patient each time it is administered. Complications can range from the inconsequential and temporary to the serious and permanent, even death in extreme cases. Some of the complications that the doctor will probably discuss with you are: heavy bleeding and scarring, nerve injury and paralysis, infection, allergic reactions, skin or hair loss and excess pigment formation. If we are frightening you with these words of caution, it's because we want you to go into plastic surgery with your eyes wide open. You must gather the information and make an informed decision as to whether the expected results from your procedure outweigh the possible risks, however remote they may be.

Almost every plastic surgeon is going to want you to sign a form consenting to surgery, stating that you have been informed that there is the possibility of complications and you wish to proceed with the operation, fully aware of the risks. This consent form may range from a long detailed document full of fine print to a fairly simple form written in simple language. In view of the booming business of malpractice attorneys, it's easy to understand the doctor's effort to protect himself and you. This entire process is called **INFORMED CONSENT**. Most of the doctors that we interviewed came up with some version similar to this definition of Informed Consent: **The patient has a reasonable understanding of the procedure along with its risks and complications as well as a realistic expectation of the anticipated results.** Here are some of the items that you can expect to be included in your surgeon's Informed Consent Form:

- A brief description of the type of procedure
- Date of surgery
- Acknowledgement of risks, and agreement that risks and complications have been discussed and that they are understood.
- Consent to use anesthesia
- Name of person to administer anesthesia
- Acknowledgment that results are not guaranteed
- Statement that information provided by you in your medical history are true and complete.
- Agreement to follow preoperative and postoperative instructions
- Permission to take "before and after" photographs and to use them in a manner specified at a later date.

You should read the form carefully and sign *only* after you completely understand all of the information contained within it.

WHERE WILL MY PROCEDURE BE PERFORMED?

Cosmetic surgery is generally performed in one of three different types of medical facilities: a hospital, an outpatient surgical center or the doctor's own

 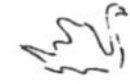

surgical center. Where your procedure will be done may depend on what type of surgery you're scheduling, what facilities the surgeon has available and, in some cases, what type of anesthesia will be necessary for your operation. Even a plastic surgeon with his own on-site surgical facility may elect to perform your surgery at a hospital if he feels the circumstances warrant that type of medical environment.

As a rule, the costs for a procedure done in a hospital are higher than those for a procedure that the surgeon can do either in his own surgical facility or at an outpatient center. The reasons are obvious - the additional expenses that the hospital will charge for your care. Again, the doctor may be in favor of a hospital setting even in light of the additional expense, especially if your procedure will require someone to monitor your immediate post-operative recovery for a period of more than a few hours.

Some hospitals have outpatient or "ambulatory" surgical facilities available. These centers are usually more relaxed in atmosphere and have a less "clinical" feel than the hospital itself, but still provide the comfort of immediate emergency care if it is needed. These facilities are an option for procedures that do not require an overnight stay for post-operative monitoring. The cost is usually less than if the procedure is done in the hospital itself.

Lastly, your plastic surgeon may have a surgical facility in his offices. If this is the case with your doctor, you should make certain that the facilities meet state standards and includes the following:

- Qualified staffing, to include a registered nurse and properly certified anesthetist.
- Patient monitoring and emergency equipment such as an EKG monitor, oxygen source, resuscitation equipment and emergency power source.

Feel free to question the doctor or his staff about the certification of their on-site surgical facility.

ANESTHESIA

Very few people (much less prospective surgery patients) realize the important part that the anesthesiologist plays in the surgical process. If you're like most people, you probably assume that this person merely comes in prior to the procedure and "puts you to sleep". Nothing could be further from the truth. The fact is that the anesthesiologist is a medical specialist who, while in the operating room, has the ultimate authority over and responsibility for the well-being of the patient. This physician will make the decision, along with input from the surgeon and the patient, on the type and strength of anesthesia that will be used prior to and during the surgery. In the operating room the anesthesiologist will monitor, among other things, the patient's heart and respiratory rate, blood pressure,

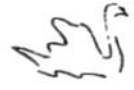

muscle movement and fluid levels. After surgery the anesthesiologist will assure that the patient recovers adequately from the anesthetics.

Each plastic surgery procedure is unique in what type of anesthetic will be used and who will administer that medication. As a rule, one (or more) of three people will handle the anesthesia for your procedure: a physician anesthesiologist, a nurse anesthetist, or the plastic surgeon himself. The type and scope of the procedure, general health of the patient, the length of time that the surgery is expected to take and surgeon/patient preference are some of the factors which will determine what type of anesthetic will be administered and by whom. A physician anesthesiologist is a medical doctor who has specialized in this branch of medicine, and has completed a residency prior to board certification. A nurse anesthetist is generally a certified registered nurse who has the standard four year nursing degree and has received specialized and on-the-job training in anesthesia.

Some procedures, such as breast reduction and nose reshaping, are commonly done with general anesthesia under the administration of a physician anesthesiologist. Other types of plastic surgery are routinely performed utilizing a combination of heavy sedation and local anesthesia under the direction of a physician anesthesiologist or a nurse anesthetist. More minor procedures such as mole removal may utilize only a local anesthetic given by the plastic surgeon himself.

General anesthesia places the patient in a state of unconsciousness. Most of us think of this as being "asleep" during the operation; we are, in fact, in a condition that is much deeper and more profound than your regular night-time sleep. Under general anesthesia, the patient is totally unaware of what is happening and will not feel any physical sensation associated with the surgery. If you and your surgeon determine that you will be under general anesthesia for your procedure, this is what you can expect to happen prior to surgery:

1. The anesthesiologist will ask you some pertinent questions such as the condition of your general health, any known allergies or chronic conditions, if you smoke or are taking any medications and any previous experiences with anesthetics. *It is very important to answer completely and honestly!*
2. After the anesthesiologist has finished your pre-operative screening, feel free to ask any questions that you may have regarding the anesthetic process. The anesthesiologists that we interviewed said that the most common patient question was "Will I be asleep or awake?" The answer, of course, will depend on the type of anesthesia that will be administered. Talk to your anesthesiologist - he or she will most likely give you a great deal of reassurance and sooth your pre-operative nerves!
3. Medication may be given at this point to relieve your anxiety, and you could be given something to inhibit excess salivation. (Remember all the

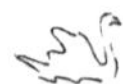

stories you've heard about "dry mouth" after surgery? This is the culprit - but it's very important for your safety!)

4. After you're feeling relaxed from the medication a tube may be inserted into a vein in your arm or wrist. This is used so that other medications can be administered very rapidly throughout the surgery.

5. If your anesthesia will be induced or maintained using gases, the mask will probably be placed over your nose and mouth now. Some general anesthetics used for plastic surgery procedures allow the patient to breath on their own; others require mechanical devices be used to assist breathing. The most common method of artifical respiration is to insert a tube in the patient's mouth and into the throat to provide air to the lungs.

6. Good night! By this point, you're probably drifting into a unconscious state and surgery will soon begin.

Throughout the surgery the anesthesiologist will be monitoring your vital signs and keeping a close eye on you to make sure you're doing well. After the surgery is complete, the anesthesiologist will monitor your immediate postoperative recovery. With general anesthesia, waking up is a slow process. As a rule, the longer the surgery, the longer the anesthetic recovery period. It will vary by patient, but usually within forty-five to ninety minutes after surgery you'll begin to be aware of what is going on. Post-operative pain medication will also be a factor in how long it takes for you to become fully cognizant. In addition to observing your state of awareness, the anesthesiologist will make sure that you are able to hold down liquids and that any nausea or dizziness has passed before he or she releases you from his care. If you are not staying overnight in a medically supervised environment, the anesthesiologist will probably advise you to be in the company of a responsible adult for at least twenty-four hours and not to sign any legally binding documents for up to forty-eight hours following the use of general anesthesia. Obviously, you should not be driving or operating any machinery for that same period. Usually, you will not be ready to go home any sooner than three hours after surgery.

As we have stressed in other sections of the first two chapters of this book, surgery and anesthesia are not without risk and possible complication. The most common complications of general anesthesia are post-operative nausea and vomiting, sore throat, and dryness of the mouth. Anesthesiologists usually try to prevent these common complications with medication. Other more serious complications are fairly rare, but you must be aware that the risk exists for: chipped teeth, dehydration, fever, allergic reaction, aspiration (inhaling vomit into the lungs), heart attack, stroke and even death. By all means, discuss these risks and possible complications with your surgeon and anesthesiologist!

Local anesthesia, sometimes combined with heavy sedation, is another option that your surgeon may recommend for your procedure. Many plastic

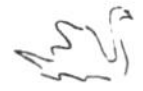

surgeons will offer this type of anesthetic to a patient as an alternative to general anesthesia due to cost factors (it is usually less expensive than general anesthesia), if the patient is wary of the possible complications of general anesthesia, or if the procedure just doesn't warrant being placed into an unconscious state. Again, this type of anesthesia may be administered by a physician anesthesiologist, but some plastic surgeons may have a nurse anesthetist on his staff who is qualified to administer these medications. Be sure to find out before surgery who will be handling your anesthesia. If you are uncomfortable with the surgeon's choice or if you have specific health concerns, ask for other options. If a local anesthetic combined with sedation medication is selected for use in your procedure, this is what you can expect immediately prior to surgery:

1. The anesthetist, nurse or surgeon will question you on your medical history, allergies, etc.
2. Be sure to take this opportunity to discuss with the anesthetist the type of anesthesia to be used as well as the risks and complications to be considered.
3. You will probably be given an injection of medication to relax you now, and the intravenous tube will be placed into your arm or wrist for the rapid administration of medications throughout surgery.
4. A heavy sedative is administered as an "IV drip" into the tube placed in your arm.
5. You will very quickly drift out of awareness, though you are not truly unconscious. Most likely, you will be so heavily sedated that you "nap" throughout the procedure. Sedatives will not block physical discomfort or pain, so a local anesthetic will be given now.
6. The local anesthetic will most likely be administered by injection directly into the region of the body that will be affected by the surgery. Depending on the anesthetic used, the surgeon may wait a few minutes for the medication to interrupt the nerve actions that relate to pain. Your local anesthetic may also include medication such as adrenaline, which is used to decrease bleeding during surgery.
7. The surgery commences, with the anesthetist monitoring the condition and state of awareness of the patient. If necessary, the level of sedation may be adjusted to keep the patient comfortable throughout the surgery.
8. Once the surgery is complete, the intravenous sedation will be discontinued. The patient will regain full awareness relatively slowly once the medication is stopped.

Once again, the anesthetist will monitor the immediate postoperative recovery of the patient to assure that all goes well when coming out from under

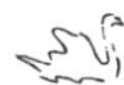

sedation. The patient may continue to feel a little "groggy", and full awareness will return gradually with this type of anesthesia. As with most types of anesthesia, a period of quiet, supervised rest is advised, even if the patient will be released from the surgical center and will not be monitored by medical personnel in the hours after recovery. Again, driving and other activities that require a clear mind and keen reflexes should be avoided for at least twenty-four hours after surgery.

Even though under local anesthesia the patient will not lose consciousness, there are risks and complications that need to be understood prior to surgery. A patient can have an adverse reaction to the medication if too heavy a dose is administered, if the medication is too rapidly absorbed by the body, or if the patient is allergic to the medication. Complications relating to these types of reactions can be nausea, dizziness, loss of consciousness, long term nerve damage, seizures, or even heart attack. In addition, any time the surface of the skin is permeated, the risk of infection exists. These risks may be rare, but *must be known and understood prior to consent to surgery.*

A final note on medications: your surgeon or anesthesiologist may recommend that you discontinue use of some drugs prior to your surgery. Aspirin and aspirin-containing products can thin the blood, and the doctor may advise that you stop using them up to two weeks prior to surgery. Any prescription drugs that are intended to thin the blood will fall into that same category. Lastly, if you are on any prescription antidepressant drugs you should discuss this use with your surgeon and anesthesiologist during your consultation and prior to surgery.

Hopefully, you now have a better understanding of the part that anesthesia and your anesthesiologist will play in your plastic surgery. You should discuss with your plastic surgeon and his staff what type of anesthesia will be used, the risks and complications involved, who will be administering your anesthesia and what their qualifications are. *Don't be shy about asking these questions*! Ask the doctor about your options in regard to anesthesia, and about certification of the medical personnel who will be handling it in your case.

HOW MUCH WILL IT COST?

At some point during the consultation process, the doctor - or more likely - someone on his staff will discuss with you what all of this will cost. You should not leave the office, and more importantly, not schedule surgery until you have a thorough understanding of the expense involved for your procedure, as well as fees for any anesthesia and post-operative care that will be necessary. Prices may differ according to geographic area, how much work will be required by the surgeon during the operation, and where the surgery will take place. Be sure to read the section in this chapter subtitled "*Where Will My Procedure Be Performed?*" That section

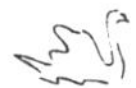

goes into greater detail about the types of surgical facilities commonly used by plastic surgeons. Be certain that you understand the total expected cost of your procedure, including fees to be charged by the anesthesiologist.

The following chart reflects data collected by the ASPRS from its members on the range of surgeon's fees charged for cosmetic procedures performed in 1990. More detailed information on the fees charged for a specific procedure and where (hospital, outpatient clinic, etc.) that procedure is most commonly performed will appear in the chapter of this book devoted to that type of surgery.

AVERAGE SURGEON'S FEE RANGES FOR COSMETIC PROCEDURES IN 1990

Procedure	Fee Range
FACELIFT	$1200 - $8000
BREAST ENLARGEMENT	$1000 - $5500
NOSE RESHAPING	$300 - $6000
BREAST REDUCTION	$1500 - $8000
EYELID SURGERY (Uppers & Lowers)	$1000 - $5000
BREAST LIFT	$1000 - $6500
TUMMY TUCK	$1200 - $8500
CHEMICAL PEEL (Full Face)	$500 - $3000
LIPOSUCTION (For any single site)	$500 - $5000
FOREHEAD LIFT	$1000 - $4000
COLLAGEN INJECTIONS (by cubic centimeter injected)	$100 - $500
CHIN IMPLANT	$300 - $2500

Fees differ substantially throughout specific geographic regions of the country. As a rule, the fees on the coasts are higher than those found in the interior areas of the United States. A doctor's fees should not be your primary deciding

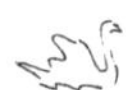

factor in choosing a surgeon; weigh credentials and experience over price in your selection process.

HOW WILL I PAY FOR MY PROCEDURE?

Aesthetic plastic surgery (an operation undertaken to improve appearance) is considered an *elective* operation, and therefore not generally covered by health insurance. In some cases involving procedures such as breast reduction or eyelid surgery, the condition may be contributing to a medical problem and the insurance company may work with you on covering all or part of the surgical expense. If you feel that this may be the case in your situation, you would be wise to discuss this option with your surgeon as well as the insurance company **prior** to scheduling the operation.

In purely cosmetic procedures, the burden of expense will probably fall entirely on you and your pocketbook. In our interviews with plastic surgery patients we found that most people had been saving money to pay for their procedure, just as they would save for any other major purchase. We found that a few patients had elected to take a cash advance on a major bank credit card or even apply for a personal loan at their bank or credit union to cover the costs. Whatever means you elect to utilize to pay the expenses, be aware that the surgeon generally will want payment in advance of the day of surgery. This is entirely reasonable, considering that he or she will probably "block out" up to an entire day on his schedule to devote to your surgery.

If an anesthesiologist will be used for your procedure the cost is usually separate from that of the surgeon. Be certain to find out the extent of this expense prior to scheduling surgery.

SUMMING IT UP

You should walk away from your initial consultation with your plastic surgeon fully confident with the ability and credentials of everyone that's to be involved in your procedure. If you aren't 100 percent sure or if you still have a great deal of apprehension following this visit, we heartily encourage you to identify the source of your concern. If it is with the surgeon and his staff, you may want to schedule a consultation with the second plastic surgeon on your list of qualified candidates. If you are confused about some of the issues covered in the consultation, go home and make a list of questions and call the doctor's office in a day or so and discuss them with the surgeon or his staff. Make sure to read the chapter in this book that is devoted to the type of procedure that you're considering. If you have doubts or concerns about anesthesia, call the anesthesiologist's office.

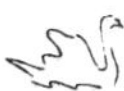

Finally, if you are questioning the wisdom of even considering plastic surgery, give it all a few days to sink in. You've had a lot of information thrown at you in this first visit, and it can be overwhelming. Think things over and discuss the issue with your spouse, parent or close friend. Plastic surgery is permanent, and everyone involved wants you to make a sound, well-informed decision.

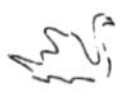

CHAPTER THREE

EYELID SURGERY

"When the eyes say one thing, and the tongue another, a practised man relies on the language of the first."

Emerson
"*Behavior*," *The Conduct of Life* (1860)

Perhaps more than any other facial feature, our eyes seem to have a way of conveying our outlook on life. If we're tired, sick or upset, our eyes let the world know. Virtually every book that you happen to pick up on effective communication and body language advises you to look someone in the eye to establish firm contact and to assist in reading the reactions of the person to whom you're speaking. But what if our eyes are sending a message to the world that just isn't accurate? What if you have drooping upper eyelids that may seem to others as though you're disinterested, bored or just not "tuned in"? What if you have puffy bags under your eyes that others might interpret, even subconsciously, as signs of fatigue, excessive consumption of alcohol, lack of sleep or advancing age? If you are like almost one-hundred thousand of the people who found themselves facing this dilemma in 1990 alone, you may chose to undergo plastic surgery of the eyelid.

According to data gathered by the ASPRS from its members, of all cosmetic surgery procedures performed in 1990, eyelid procedures, or **blepharoplasty**, accounted for over twelve percent of the total. In addition, it was one of the most common procedures undertaken by men, second only to nose reshaping. It was the number one cosmetic procedure choice for patients aged fifty-one and over. This number of eyelid procedures represents a whopping forty percent increase over the eyelid procedures performed in 1981 by members of the same professional society.

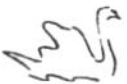

Experts cite various reasons for the dramatic increase, but many agree that the perceived pressure to compete in the career world with younger, more aggressive workers plays a part in the decision of older persons to try and present a more youthful, energetic appearance. In fact, plastic surgeons indicate that eyelid surgery can be one of the procedures that patients consider at an earlier age than any other type of cosmetic procedure.

Eyelid surgery is also one of the plastic surgery procedures that may be considered for reasons other than merely appearance. In some cases, the upper eyelid may droop to such a degree that peripheral vision is effected. In the most extreme, a "hood" is formed by the upper eyelid, folding over itself beneath the eyebrow and above the eyelashes. In such instances, your plastic surgeon may recommend that you see an eye specialist (ophthamologist or optometrist) to have a visual field examination to determine if your peripheral vision has been impaired by your condition. If that situation exists, your health insurance company may pay some or all of the costs associated with the surgery. *Be sure to discuss this possibility with your plastic surgeon at the time of consultation.*

"How did this happen to me, anyway?" you ask. As usual, aging is one culprit that can generally be blamed for droopy upper eyelids and puffy bags underneath the eyes. There are other factors that could have contributed to this condition, however. Heredity (*thanks, Mom!*), excessive squinting caused by exposure to sun or cigarette smoking, allergies, and pregnancy can all help along Father Time in producing these symptoms. Because of this, senior citizens aren't the only candidates for plastic surgery of the eyelid - plastic surgeons sometimes see patients in their twenties or thirties who are viable candidates for blepharoplasty due to inherited characteristics. All of the above mentioned factors can contribute to the weakening of the membranes and muscles surrounding the eye. As the membrane and muscle weakens, fatty tissue is held less taut and therefore "bags" or "pooches out". In addition, many people can experience an accumulation of fluid in the membranes of the eye region, further weakening and stretching the tissue and causing it to lose some of its elasticity.

As these circumstances occur, the upper and lower eyelids can begin to sag and bulge to a noticeable degree. Women usually begin noticing difficulty in applying eye makeup, and both sexes may notice perspiration in the folds of the eye becoming a problem. It is at this time that some people choose to see a plastic surgeon.

WHO IS A CANDIDATE FOR EYELID SURGERY?

In general, almost anyone in good health and with the right motivation and expectations of results (see Chapters One and Two) is a good candidate for eyelid

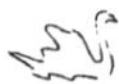

surgery if the condition exists at a degree that is correctable by surgery. As a rule, the age of the patient has little impact on the prospects for good results in the eyelid procedure. In addition, the results of the surgery are usually extremely long-lasting. Your plastic surgeon will, of course, do a full evaluation of your condition at the time of consultation. Some of the things that he or she will be looking at are:

- Your overall health
- Wrinkles
- Muscle tone
- Glasses/Contact Lenses
- Skin Elasticity
- Skin type
- Amount of fat to be removed
- Visual problems/Glaucoma
- Amount of normal eye tearing
- Asymmetry of eyes and eyebrows

Most surgeons will check to see if you have "dry eyes", since that condition may be aggravated by blepharoplasty. If you think that this applies to you, be certain to discuss it with your surgeon.

In some cases, it may be recommended that the eyelid procedure be combined with a forehead or eyebrow lift. Since these procedures are most commonly associated with a facelift, we will include a brief explanation of forehead and eyebrow lifts in the chapter devoted to facelifts.

Fine lines and wrinkles around the eye may be best treated with a light to medium chemical peel after the blepharoplasty. Discuss this with your surgeon and read Chapter Eleven for more detail.

PREOPERATIVE INSTRUCTIONS

At the time that you schedule your procedure, either the doctor or someone on his staff will review with you some instructions that you should follow in the days or weeks immediately prior to your surgery, as well as for the day that your procedure is to be done. Some of the more common items that most surgeons will include are:

- Do not take any medication containing aspirin for up to two weeks prior to surgery (can cause excessive bleeding).
- The surgeon may recommend that the patient take additional Vitamin C for a few days prior to surgery.
- Stop cigarette smoking: affects healing and may cause skin loss in facelifts and other procedures.
- No alcoholic beverages up to forty-eight hours prior to surgery.
- Nothing to eat or drink after midnight the night before surgery.

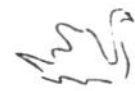

- **Irregularities in the lower eyelid**: such as a small bulge or depressed area can be noticable after healing. Bulges are present if a small amount of localized fat remains under the skin; depressed areas are caused by an irregularity in the amount of fat removed during surgery. Both of the above may require secondary surgery to correct.

These are *some* of the risks and complications that must be considered when undergoing eyelid surgery. The list is by no means complete and is expressed in generalities only. You **must** discuss risks and complications with your surgeon and his staff, and be fully aware of the possibility of these risks, as well as other complications that may not be detailed in this book. **Your best defense against the vast majority of these risks and complica-tions is to schedule your surgery with a qualified surgeon experienced in eyelid surgery.** Our aim in this book is to give you the information that will help you make an informed, responsible decision.

COST

All of the statistics mentioned in this section are based on information gathered by the American Society of Plastic and Reconstructive Surgeons for procedures performed by their members in 1990. In that year, over ninety percent of the eyelid procedures were performed on an outpatient basis, meaning that a hospital stay was not necessary for these patients. Bear in mind that these fees are averages only, and that the costs of your procedure may vary widely from these figures. Fees differ throughout the geographic regions of the country, and even in cities within the same state. The average surgeon's fees for the eyelid procedure in 1990 were:

LOW	AVERAGE	HIGH
$1000	$2450	$5000

THE EYELID PROCEDURE

Blepharoplasty (eyelid surgery) is performed for the purpose of tightening and removing excess skin and fat from the upper and/or lower eyelids. This redundant skin and fatty tissue causes the upper lids to droop and lower eyelids to "bag". Surgery is commonly performed on both the upper and lower lids during the same session, and is **not** usually done in an effort to eliminate wrinkles. Excess wrinkling in the region of the eye is generally handled with other cosmetic

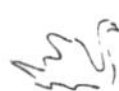

procedures, such as the chemical peel.

The upper eyelids are almost always done first. The doctor may use a small measuring device (called calipers) on your upper lid to measure the amount of skin and tissue that needs to be removed. The surgeon will generally make some marks directly on your eyelid to use as a guide during surgery, indicating where the incisions will be made and how much tissue will be cut away. The incisions will be made within the natural crease of the eyelid, and will extend to the outer corner of the eye into the "crow's feet" wrinkles. The width of the incision will depend on the amount of skin that needs to be removed.

The surgeon will then remove the skin that lies within the incision, followed by the removal of the underlying excess fatty tissue. Once he is satisfied that all the necessary skin, fat and tissue have been removed, he will close the incision with the type and number of sutures (stitches) he deems appropriate. If you are having both upper and lower lids done, the surgeon will now begin on the lower lid.

The surgery on the lower eyelid is the part of the procedure which calls most heavily on the expertise and experience of the surgeon. If too much skin or fatty tissue is removed, the patient can experience permanent ectropion, where the lower lid no longer lies flush against the eyeball, and may have a marked "pull down" appearance that exposes an unusual amount of the white in the lower half of the eye. The surgeon will make the lower incision just below the edge of the eyelashes, again extending out into the fine wrinkles at the outside corner of the eye. The extra skin, muscle and fatty tissue that are producing the unsightly bags and pouches is then removed and the incision is closed.

The procedure will most likely take from one to three hours, depending on whether both lids are done, the amount of bleeding, and how extensive the surgery. Your surgeon may choose to apply small tape strips or dressings on the eye. Some surgeons will have cold compresses applied to the eyes immediately following surgery to help alleviate swelling, bruising and discomfort. The doctor may release you within a few hours and your chauffeur for the day can drive you home. Remember to have a responsible adult at your disposal for at least twenty-four hours!

If you have chosen your surgeon carefully and follow his postoperative instructions, the small scars made by these incisions should completely heal within a couple of months. In a successful eyelid procedure, the scars are scarcely visible and the results can be dramatic.

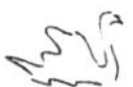

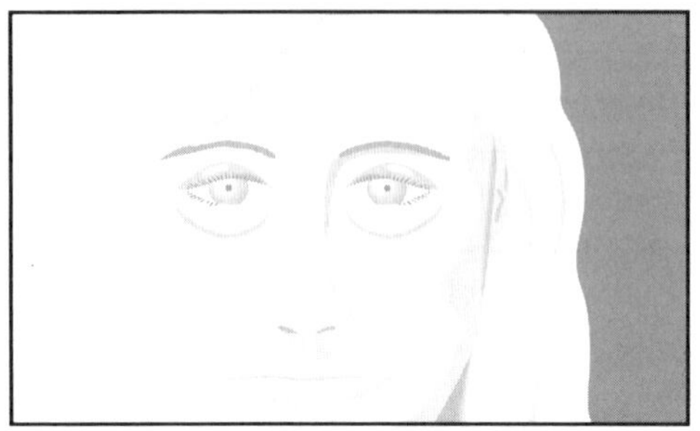

Preoperative eyelid patient with excess skin and baggy upper and lower eyelids.

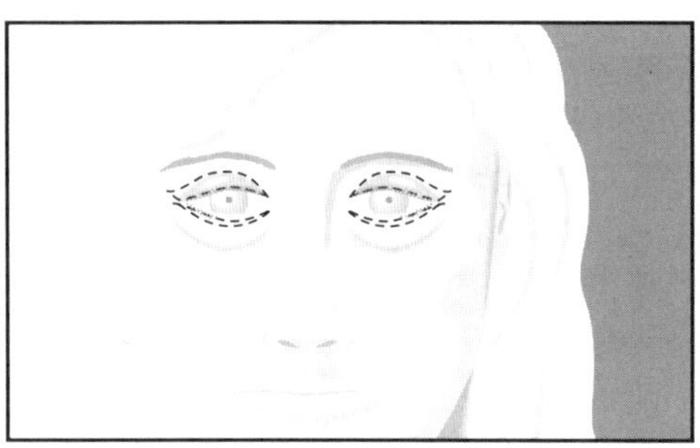

Lines showing the location of incisions commonly made for eyelid surgery. The skin between the dotted lines will be removed.

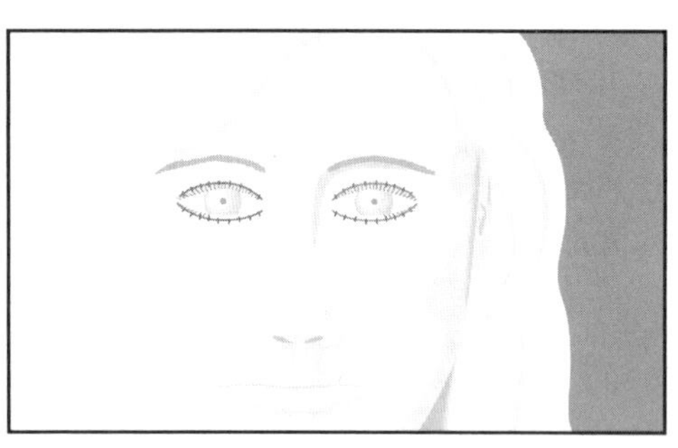

These lines represent the tiny sutures that are used to close the incisions made on the upper and lower eyelids.

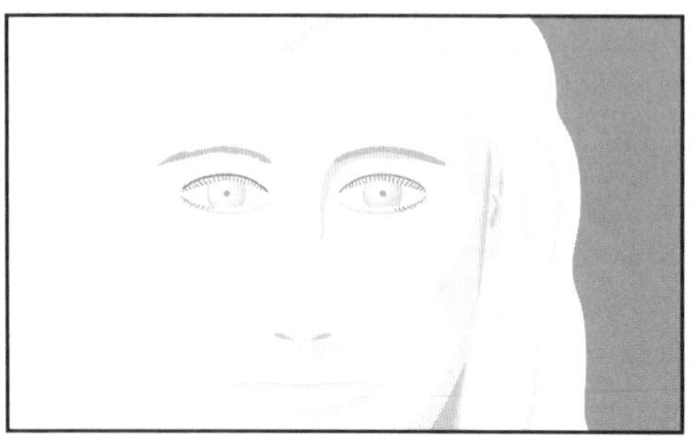

The postoperative patient with a fresher, more youthful and well-rested appearance.

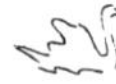

THE POSTOPERATIVE PERIOD

In the hours immediately following surgery, you may experience sensations of tightness and possibly some itching or burning in the eyelids, but rarely any serious discomfort. A mild over-the-counter pain medication should be sufficient. Any serious pain or swelling should be reported to the surgeon, since it may be an indication of bleeding. The doctor will advise you to apply ice and/or cold cloth compresses to the eye region periodically throughout the first day and up to three days following surgery. **Ice is critical** in alleviating some of the discomfort as well as diminish swelling. The doctor will probably advise you to rest for at least a day or two, and to **avoid excess talking or movement**. Strenuous activity should be avoided for up to two or three weeks. Ask you surgeon about any specific activities that you have questions about. Other postoperative instructions that the doctor may include are:

- **Elevate** the head moderately for the first few days. Rest in a recliner chair whenever convenient, and sleep on your back with two pillows supporting the head. Try to avoid bending the head down as much as possible, even when washing your hair. These precautions are needed to help alleviate swelling and prevent bleeding.
- **Medication** may be given to apply directly into the eye. This is to help relieve the dryness (and subsequent redness) of the eye. Some patients may need some form of "artificial tears" for up to a few weeks after surgery.
- **Scars** are probably a major concern to you right now. Be aware that scars go through a couple of stages in the healing process: at first, the incisions may be barely noticeable. After a short interval, the scars may become red and "angry looking" for a period of time. In as soon as a few weeks or up to a few months after surgery, your scars should mature into fine lines that are scarcely visible. After the initial recovery period and when approved by your doctor, makeup can be used to help hide any noticeable scarring. Some doctors allow the careful application of makeup within three or four days after surgery.
- **Bruising** is to be expected for the first couple of weeks. Be aware that not every patient heals at the same rate. Your bruises may disappear very quickly, or may persist for longer than a couple of weeks. Light colored bruises will clear more quickly than blackish bruises, and older patients tend to bruise more extensively due to thinner skin. Warm compresses applied after swelling goes away will help the bruises to fade.
- **Swelling** is also to be anticipated for at least a week following surgery, possibly longer. This can prevent you from being able to close your eyes completely for a few days, hence the dryness and irritation to the eye itself.

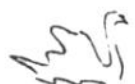

YOU SHOULD IMMEDIATELY REPORT ANY EXCESSIVE OR RAPID SWELLING TO YOUR SURGEON!

- **Bandages** are not generally neccessary with this procedure.
- **Sutures** (stitches) are usually taken out within 2 to 3 days after surgery. Your doctor will place small strips of tape across the outer lower lid after surgery, to be removed when the sutures are taken out. If necessary, the tape may be reapplied for support.
- **Alcohol** intake will be restricted for the first week.
- **Sunglasses** will be recommended for a week or two following surgery, especially when going out. The purpose is two-fold: to keep dust and other irritants out of the eye and incisions, and to protect the already sensitive eye from the harsh glare of sunlight (and from the curious looks from people reacting to your bruises and swelling!).
- **Sunburn** should always be avoided - whether you've had cosmetic surgery or not. Exposure to the sun may be limited by your doctor for a period.
- **Makeup** will probably be permitted after the first few days if you're healing properly.
- **Contact lenses** may be uncomfortable for a period of time following surgery due to swelling and tenderness of the eye region. We advise that you discuss this issue directly with your surgeon and/or eye specialist.

You'll probably be looking fairly normal within ten days to two weeks after surgery. Your doctor may indicate that you can return to work, with certain precautions, after as few as four or five days. *You should follow **your** surgeon's postoperative instructions very closely, and question the doctor or his staff on any specific issues that are not addressed in his standard guidelines.* The items we mention here are, again, generalities. Any instructions given to you by your surgeon should supercede those outlined in this chapter.

We'd like to mention at this point something that patients may experience after a plastic surgery procedure - *a mild and temporary postoperative depression.* Don't let it worry you if you feel slightly discouraged or disappointed with yourself and your surgical results in the first few days after the procedure is performed. You're bruised, swollen and maybe a little uncomfortable. You may be even questioning the wisdom of your actions because you probably look worse than you did when you first walked into the surgeon's office! Relax, this should soon pass. The discoloration and puffy condition of your eyes will soon diminish, as will those negative feelings that you may be experiencing. If you are truly troubled, call and talk to the doctor or someone on his staff.

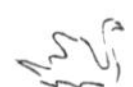

RESULTS

The results of blepharoplasty, as we have mentioned before, can be dramatic. Some plastic surgeons go so far as to state that eyelid surgery can do more to improve the youthful appearance of a patient than any other type of cosmetic procedure. Particularly if the condition of the eyelids prior to surgery was affecting vision, the results of this procedure often absolutely delight the patients who undergo the surgery. Since the effects of eyelid surgery are long-lasting (usually at least a dozen to fifteen years), some patients feel as if eyelid procedures are the "bargains" in the cosmetic surgery goody-bag.

As indicated previously, the eyelid procedure is intended to tighten the skin around the eye and to reduce drooping or baggy eyelids. This procedure, as a rule, will not go very far in reducing the number of wrinkles in your face. Other cosmetic procedures such as facelifts, forehead or brow lifts and chemical peels may be necessary if you are looking for more than the eyelid procedure can do for you.

In addition, plastic surgery of the eyelid will **not**, as a rule, change the shape or expression of your eyes. Those persons with an Oriental appearance through heredity have some option open to them in creating a more rounded eye, but this should be thought out carefully and discussed thoroughly with the surgeon in consultation.

Patience is of the upmost importance before judging the permanent results of your cosmetic surgery. A very few blepharoplasty patients may experience a temporary or (in rare instances) permanent "wide-eyed" look after surgery. Discuss this issue with your surgeon.

As with all cosmetic procedures, you should choose your surgeon carefully. Verification of credentials and level of experience is essential, since eyelid surgery requires a great deal of experience, skill and expertise to produce pleasing results.

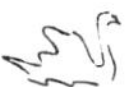

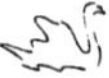

CHAPTER FOUR

THE FACELIFT PROCEDURE

"If eyes were made for seeing, then Beauty is its own excuse for being."

Emerson
"*Beauty*" *The Conduct of Life* (1860)

The facelift, or ***rhytidectomy***, is the one procedure that most people readily associate with cosmetic or plastic surgery. In the not so distant past, many perceived cosmetic surgery as a medical convenience existing primarily to provide facelifts for wealthy socialites, actresses and other public figures who were making an attempt to reverse the tell-tale visible signs of advancing age. As we have discussed in this book, there are large numbers of plastic surgery procedures undertaken for purely *aesthetic* (to improve the appearance) purposes by all types of people for all kinds of reasons. The fact is, according to data gathered by the ASPRS from its members, facelifts rank sixth in the list of all cosmetic procedures performed by members in 1990.

The almost fifty thousand facelifts done in 1990 by members of that society alone represented a twenty-five percent increase over the number of facelifts done in 1981, with over ninety percent of those procedures being undertaken by women. The majority (fifty-nine percent) of those patients range from fifty-one to sixty-four years old, and another twenty-seven percent are between the ages of thirty-five and fifty.

Interviews with facelift patients reveal a variety of reasons for electing to undergo the procedure: displeasure with appearance almost always plays a part in choosing a facelift, as does the desire for a more youthful countenance. Perhaps not surprisingly, a number of patients refer to career related issues as being at least a slight factor in considering a facelift. Some employees are facing keen competition

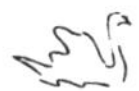

from younger, more aggressive co-workers and feel that a more youthful appearance can only help in maintaining a competitive edge in the career market.

In addition to the pressures of the workplace, our society itself places no small amount of emphasis on the benefits and desirability of a youthful appearance. Television, the print media and product advertising all tend to focus on the premise that "younger is better". Even those among us who are comfortable with a few wrinkles, laugh lines and a random pouch of cellulite or two may consider altering their appearance to conform with society's ideal of a perpetually youthful face, body and lifestyle. We are bombarded with a constant barrage of advertising to look younger, feel younger and think younger. In the face of this pressure, a large number of people each year are utilizing the medical means available to help diminish the visible signs of aging.

The medical term for facelift is **rhytidectomy**, which is latin for *wrinkle* **(rhytid)** *removal* **(ectomy)**. The term *facelift* is in itself somewhat misleading, since the procedure also places a focus on the area beneath the chin and in the upper neck. The primary benefit of a facelift is the improvement of deep wrinkles and sagging tissues of the face and neck, with the key word being **improvement**. This is accomplished by the removal of excess skin and fat, as well as the tightening of sagging muscles. The facelift procedure, by itself, will not generally diminish any wrinkling around the lips, in the forehead or eyelids, or at the base of the neck. These problem areas may require additional procedures such as eyelid surgery (blepharoplasty), forehead and/or brow lift and the use of chemical peels. Liposuction (fat suctioning) is also sometimes used by surgeons to remove excess fatty tissue in the problem areas. The face and neck area generally appear more firm and have a smoother appearance as a result of the facelift operation.

Each person wears age in a manner uniquely their own. The condition of your face and neck, as with the rest of your body, depends on many factors, including those that are hereditary as well as environmental. Some of the culprits contributing to sagging skin, fat accumulation and loose muscle tissue in the face and neck are: heredity, age (of course), weight change and skin damage from exposure to the sun and wind. As the skin loses its elasticity, the forces of gravity contribute to sagging and wrinkling. With the passing of years, our skin also thins and dries out, further diminishing the wonderful "plumpness" that our cells enjoyed in their youth.

Just as each person ages differently, each patient will experience a varied degree of improvement from a facelift. Some patients enjoy results that are a dramatic change for the better, while others may see a less marked improvement in the face and neck. Remember, too, that a facelift will not change the natural shape of your face or neck, nor will it normally alter your facial expression. In fact, many top-notch surgeons greatly advocate the repositioning of facial fat as much as possible, rather than the wholesale removal of the fat. Dr. John R. Royer in Winter

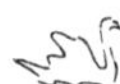

Park, Florida, emphasizes, "Removal [of facial fat] rather than restoring it to a proper position may produce a future generation of "facial anorexics" who need their fat as they age. What may appear to be excess fat in the jowls or mid-face may become nicely rounded cheekbones when restored to the original position in the face."

Your surgeon will discuss in detail what results he expects to achieve from your operation, probably during your consultation. Most patients can anticipate a face that appears anywhere from five to ten years younger, depending on the set of circumstances (age, skin elasticity, etc.) unique to that patient. Bear in mind that a facelift, no matter how successful, *does not stop the aging process*. Your face, just like the rest of you, will continue to age.

WHO IS A CANDIDATE FOR A FACELIFT?

In general, almost anyone in good health and with the right motivation and expectations of results (see Chapters One and Two) is a good candidate for a facelift. As a rule, the age of the patient has less impact on the prospects for good results in the facelift procedure than one might imagine. More important than chronological age is the condition of the skin itself, the amount of wrinkling and sagging present, skin elasticity, skin type and coloring and bone structure.

Your plastic surgeon will, of course, do a full evaluation of your condition at the time of consultation. Some of the things that he or she will be looking at are:

- Your overall health
- Skin type and coloring
- Amount of wrinkling
- Muscle tone
- Amount of fat to be removed or repositioned
- Bone structure
- Neck Angle
- Hereditary factors (race, ethnic features, etc)
- Skin Elasticity
- Damage from sun and wind exposure

While age is not the primary factor, there are certain generalities that can be made concerning a patient's age and the relative success of the facelift. For example, most surgeons agree that a facelift is probably not necessary on patients any younger than their late thirties. Patients concerned with wrinkling and sagging

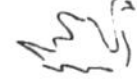

before that age may be better treated with other procedures such as the chemical peel, blepharoplasty (eyelid surgery) or the use of liposuction on fatty deposits. Most surgeons agree that the *best* results occur in patients whose ages range from the mid-forties to early fifties. Skin elasticity and bone structure are generally fairly sound within that age range, and there is usually an absence of excessive fatty deposits.

PREOPERATIVE INSTRUCTIONS

At the time that you schedule your procedure, either the doctor or someone on his staff will review with you some instructions that you should follow in the days or weeks immediately prior to your surgery, as well as for the day that your procedure is to be done. Some of the more common items that most surgeons will include are:

- Do not take any medication containing aspirin for up to two weeks prior to surgery (can cause excessive bleeding). In addition, your surgeon may recommend that you discontinue use of some hormone medications and certain vitamin supplements - check with your doctor!
- The surgeon may advise that the patient take additional Vitamin C for a few days prior to surgery, and some surgeons may prescribe an antibiotic to be taken for a specified number of days before surgery
- Stop cigarette smoking and avoid nicotine products (affects healing and may cause skin loss)
- No alcoholic beverages up to forty-eight hours prior to surgery.
- Nothing to eat or drink after midnight the night before surgery.
- Arrange for someone to drive you to and from the surgical center, as well as for a responsible adult to be with you during the first twenty-four hours or longer.
- Some tips to consider that nobody may mention: stock up on soft foods and foods that are easily chewed - you're not going to be up to rigorous chewing for the first few days after surgery. Also, purchase a good liquid oral hygiene product in case brushing your teeth is uncomfortable for a few days. Lastly, have a supply of "quiet" activities on hand to keep you busy for the first week of your recovery. Listening to music is a very good way to help you pass the time. Try to avoid excitement and visitors for the first few days.

In addition, the doctor may have you begin washing your face with special cleansing agents for a day or so prior to surgery. You may also be instructed to wash your hair the evening before surgery and to abstain from using make-up and hair

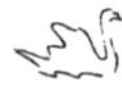

spray on surgery day. A little tidbit of advise: you may want to consider having your hair permed or colored (if you usually have those things done on a regular basis) a week or so **before** your surgery. It will be a couple of weeks, at the least, before those activities are comfortable or safe. Leave the trimming of your hair for after surgery - you may want the additional length to help hide the incisions for awhile. Be certain that you understand all of the instructions given to you; call your surgeon's office if you are confused about any of the items on his list.

ANESTHESIA

A high percentage of plastic surgeons will recommend that the facelift procedure be done at an outpatient surgical center or in his own surgical facilities. Local anesthetics combined with adequate sedation to assure the comfort of the patient may be the anesthesia of choice. These may be administered by a nurse, the doctor himself or a physician anesthesiologist. Some surgeons, due to the length of the procedure and the complexity of the operation, may advise that you undergo general anesthesia for the facelift. This allows the surgeon to concentrate on your facelift, while the physician anesthesiologist is monitoring your overall condition (blood pressure, etc). If that is the case with your operation, you will be unconscious throughout the procedure and will remember little of what transpires after the mild sedative is given to relax you prior to surgery

If your surgeon feels that local anesthesia combined with heavy sedation is adequate for your procedure, you will not be unconscious but will most likely be sedated to a degree that you "nap" throughout the operation. To remove the possibility of physical discomfort in the area of the incisions, a local anesthetic will be administered after the sedation has had time to make you relaxed. The prick of the needle and subsequent burning or stinging sensation as the local anesthetic is injected may be slightly uncomfortable, but will soon pass.

Make certain that you read Chapter Two of this book. In those pages we discuss anesthesia in detail and outline the risks and complications inherent with their use. Discuss the options with your surgeon and make certain that you are comfortable with his recommendations for the type of anesthesia **as well as with who will be administering it.**

RISKS AND COMPLICATIONS

As with any surgical procedure, there are a number of risks and complications inherent to the facelift operation. Some are minor and very common, such as bruising and swelling. Others are more serious but seen less frequently, such as an extended period of numbness in the facial area. Still other complications and risks

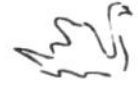

are extremely rare and very serious, such as loss of nerve function or even death. The best protection against serious complications is to choose a qualified, experienced surgeon with the skills and ability behind him that are necessary to achieve the results that you desire. This same criteria should be applied to the anesthesiologist to be used for your surgery.

As we discussed in Chapter Two, the use of some type of anesthesia is necessary for your comfort and safety in performing the facelift procedure. As with the surgery itself, there are risks and complications that accompany the use of anesthetics. Make certain to discuss these with your surgeon and anesthesiologist, and read those pages in Chapter Two again.

Some of the risks and complications that you should be aware of when considering a facelift are:

- **Bruising** should be expected, and can last to a noticeable degree up to a couple of weeks following surgery. Amount of discoloration will vary by patient, as will the length of time it takes to fade.
- **Swelling** is also very common. Obvious swelling will probably subside within a few weeks, but be aware that it may take up to as much as a few months for your face to "settle" fully after surgery. Discuss this in detail with your surgeon.
- **Bleeding** or the ***slight*** oozing of blood is not unheard of after surgery. Some surgeons may insert small "drains" to express any blood beneath the skin. Marked bleeding during or after facelift surgery is not common. *Any unusual bleeding or marked swelling of the face or neck should be immediately reported to the doctor.*
- **T*emporary* numbness** of the face is a fairly common complaint for a short time immediately after surgery, up to a few months. Some patients indicate that their face feels like a mask, followed by a period of tingling sensation that will generally signal the return of full feeling to the area. Small pockets of numbness may persist for a longer period. In unusual cases, the loss of feeling in these isolated areas is permanent.
- **Hematoma** is the pooling of blood beneath the surface of the skin, and is the most common "serious" complication of facelift surgery, in that it may require medical attention to rectify. Small hematomas may go unnoticed by the patient, since the drains inserted by the surgeon will express the excess blood. In very small hematomas, the blood may be just absorbed by the body. In other, more uncommon instances, the bleeding is more pronounced, swelling occurs and the site of the hematoma can become painful. In these unusual cases, the doctor will have to see the patient to determine the cause of the bleeding and to remove the pooled blood, probably by inserting a suction tube into the area. The surgeon may find

 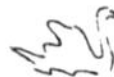

it necessary to open the incision and remove the clot. Bear in mind that this is *not* the kind of blood clot that enters your blood stream and goes to the lungs, but it *can* put pressure on the overlying skin and impair circulation, which can cause skin loss. This complication will generally occur within the first twenty-four hours following surgery (but can occur later), which is one of the reasons most surgeons will require an overnight stay with medical supervision in the initial postoperative recovery period of a facelift.

- **Skin loss** is unusual, but has occurred in patients where blood circulation in an area does not return to normal fairly rapidly. This can sometimes be attributed to an excess amount of tension on the skin in the area, an untreated hematoma, or if the patient is a smoker. The skin will generally turn a darker shade in the affected area, and will begin a peeling process similar to that following a severe sunburn. If the circulation to the area is seriously impaired, the skin may slough off and a heavy scab will form. Once the scab disappears an unsightly scar may remain. This complication is most commonly seen in the area behind the ears, where tension on the skin is usually greatest following surgery.

- **Hair loss** is fairly common. Instances of hair loss are most commonly due to an excess amount of tension on the skin in the area of the hairline incisions. When too much tension is placed on a scar it may thicken and spread, causing a loss of hair growth within the scar. A hematoma or the results of smoking can cause impaired circulation to the scalp and result in hair loss. In some cases, the hair follicles may have been damaged in the surgery process, thus causing a small area of baldness. This complication is more commonly experienced in patients undergoing subsequent facelifts rather than those who are having their first facelift. Secondary surgery for scar revision (to diminish the area of hair loss) may be possible in some patients who experience this complication.

- **Pain** following a facelift procedure is usually minimal. The surgeon may prescribe mild painkillers for the first few days following surgery, and the patient may receive injections during his or her medically supervised recovery period immediately after the operation. If severe discomfort occurs, it may be an indication of a problem requiring attention, such as a hematoma. Always report excessive pain or swelling to the surgeon.

- **Scarring** as a result of the incisions made during facelift surgery are generally well within acceptable limits to most patients. The incisions are made in inconspicuous areas such as within the hairline and in natural creases of the ear. These scars are usually barely perceptible, even without makeup. If unsightly scarring does occur, secondary surgery for purposes of scar revision may be desired.

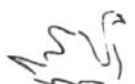

- **Infection** is very rare, but the possibility exists for this complication with any type of surgery. Your surgeon may require that you cleanse the skin and hair with special antibacterial soaps prior to surgery, as well as prescribing antibiotics to be taken for several days before your operation. Special post-operative instructions given by the doctor should be followed closely in an effort to eliminate the risk of infection.
- **Facial Nerve Injury** ranges from the temporary and inconsequential (see "Temporary Numbness", above) to the rare and permanent. In the most serious cases, a branch of the facial nerve is severed or damaged during surgery and a permanent loss of function in the lip and/or cheek muscles occurs. The eyebrow and forehead areas can also be affected, since incisions are made in the areas of those nerves as well. Cases of permanent facial nerve injury are extremely rare.

These are some of the complications and risks that the potential facelift patient must be aware of and take into consideration when making the decision to undergo the surgery. The list is by no means complete. Make certain that you discuss these and other possible complications fully with your doctor prior to signing your consent forms. Responsibility for making a well-informed decision falls on you. Plastic surgery is permanent, and should be treated as such when considering this operation.

Our intent is to give you the information that will help you make a sound, well-informed decision. If mention of the risks and complications inherent to this procedure and to anesthesia give you reason to think of this undertaking as a serious matter that can have permanent results, both positive and negative, we have accomplished our goal.

COST

The expense associated with your facelift procedure can vary to a substantial degree, depending on what type of surgical facility your plastic surgeon chooses to utilize. If your doctor feels that a hospital stay is necessary for your operation, the overall cost of your facelift will be greater than one that is done on an outpatient basis. Some facelift patients can anticipate a hospital stay of one or two days, depending on their unique situation and the recommendation of the surgeon. Most facelifts are being done on an outpatient basis; only twenty percent of the facelifts performed by members of the ASPRS in 1990 were done on an inpatient basis.

The anesthesia of choice for your operation will be a factor in your final cost, as well. General anesthesia is almost always administered by a physician

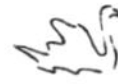

anesthesiologist whose fees are separate and above those charged by the surgeon, while local anesthesia with sedation is frequently administered by a nurse or the surgeon himself. The average surgeon's fees for facelifts done in 1990 by members of the American Society of Plastic and Reconstructive Surgeons were:

LOW	AVERAGE	HIGH
$1200	**$3880**	**$8000**

You should be aware that surgeon's fees will differ throughout geographic regions of the country. In general, prices are somewhat higher on the east and west coasts, with the least expensive procedures available in the interior regions of the United States. These are generalities and should not be used to measure the fees charged by your surgeon. Make certain that you discuss all of the costs involved for your procedure prior to surgery day, including anesthesiologist fees, post-operative care, etc.

As with most cosmetic procedures, the cost of a facelift is not usually covered by health insurance. Most surgeons will want payment of their fees prior to surgery. If your operation is to be performed in a hospital, separate arrangements may be necessary to cover those expenses. Discuss this in detail with your surgeon's staff.

THE FACELIFT PROCEDURE

In a facelift, incisions are made in front of and behind the ears, on the scalp within the hairline and behind the chin (see the illustrations). The surgeon will work on one side of the face at a time, with the work to be duplicated on the opposite side. The surgeon will separate the facial skin from the underlying fat and muscle, removing excess fat and muscle and altering position of tissue as needed. The newest techniques, however, involve a deeper dissection of facial tissue in that the surgeon works *below* the facial muscle layer. Surgeons using this technique feel it enables them to acheive a better, longer-lasting result. Some surgeons also utilize liposuction (fat suctioning) during facelifts to remove the excess fat from the cheek, jaw and neck areas. Once the removing and repositioning of tissue is complete, he will tighten and drape the skin over the facial contours.

It is very important to discuss with your plastic surgeon exactly what will be done during your surgery. The doctor may recommend that certain procedures be combined into your operation, in addition to the facelift itself. Some doctors consider these procedures to be a part of the facelift operation, others do not. The procedures most commonly done along with a facelift are the brow lift and the

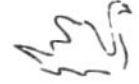

forehead lift, which we will describe briefly in this chapter. If your surgeon feels that your eyelids are in need of work, he will usually discuss the blepharoplasty procedure with you at the time of consultation. You and your surgeon may elect to do both the eyelid procedure and the facelift in the same surgical session. Be sure to read Chapter Three on the eyelid procedure if you are to undergo the eyelid procedure as well as the facelift.

When you first arrive at the hospital or surgical center, you will probably have your blood pressure and pulsed checked and have a brief interview with the anesthesiologist or nurse. These questions are to double-check what you've already indicated on your medical history: do you have any known allergies or chronic health conditions, do you smoke, etc. After everyone is satisfied that you are in a satisfactory physical condition to undergo the surgery, you may be given medication to help you relax. Also included in the preparation process is the careful trimming of hair from the incision sites on the scalp. The surgeon carefully measures the areas to be trimmed in order to assure that no shaved areas will be obvious after surgery.

Once in the operating room, you will be hooked up to monitors to keep an eye on your vital signs during surgery. An intravenous tube may be placed in your arm or wrist for sedation and any other medications that may be necessary throughout your operation. After a few minutes you will begin to feel very drowsy and relaxed. Your face will be cleansed thoroughly in preparation for surgery. If you are to be placed under general anesthesia, it will probably be administered now.

At this point the surgeon will begin marking your face, scalp and neck with a surgical pen. These marks are his "roadmap", and will help him determine how much skin can safely be detached from the underlying layers of fat and muscle. Once all his lines and arrows are in place, you will be injected with local anesthetics in the areas to be affected during surgery.

After your face is sufficiently numbed, the surgeon will begin making his incisions. Some doctors will start with the small cut to be made underneath and behind the chin. Through this incision the surgeon will work with the platysma muscle which runs from the face, down the neck and into the area of the collarbone. The doctor will tighten this muscle, creating a crisper neckline and diminish the "double chin" in the process. Be aware, however, that the surgeon will not be able to alter the natural "angle" of your neckline. If you have a sloping neckline rather than one with more of a right angle, you will have an *improved* sloping neckline after surgery.

The surgeon will now make the incisions that will enable him to smooth the excess skin and fat from your face. The incisions will be made in inconspicuous areas, such as within the hairline and in the groove behind the ear, as well as in front of the ear along the natural crease. Once the incisions are made, the doctor will

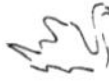

separate the skin and a thin layer of fat from the bony and muscular structure of the face. At this point, the facial skin is essentially a flap, through which the surgeon will reposition and/or remove the unwanted fat and redundant muscle tissue that is contributing to the bags, sags and jowls of the facial area.

When the excess tissue is removed, the skin is repositioned over the facial contours, being pulled taut to eliminate the previously sagging areas. Careful draping is critical in avoiding an "over operated" look that can be noticeable, even to strangers. The surgeon will probably make temporary sutures to hold the newly draped skin in position as he trims away the excess. Once the surgeon is satisfied that all redundant tissue has been trimmed away, the temporary stitches will be replaced with the sutures used to close the incision.

Throughout the facelift the doctor will be dealing with bleeding. He will be using an electrical device called a *cautery* to seal the blood vessels. In addition, most surgeons will also install small "suction drains" under the facial skin to help remove any excess bleeding and reduce bruising that occurs after the incisions are closed.

Once the surgeon's work has been done on both sides of the face, he or she may apply dressings or bandages. Some surgeons don't bandage to any great extent - they feel that bandages may prevent the detection of some post-operative complications, such as hematoma.

The entire facelift procedure will generally take anywhere from three to four hours. If additional procedures are to be done, the time in surgery can exceed five or more hours.

OTHER PROCEDURES COMMONLY DONE WITH A FACELIFT

As we mentioned before, there are a couple of procedures that frequently accompany a facelift. Be sure to discuss with your surgeon which, if any, additional procedures will be done during your surgery.

The **forehead or brow lift** is undertaken to diminish the deep furrows in the forehead, the pronounced vertical lines between the eyes and the "smile lines" found at the outer eye. This procedure will produce results that are not fully achievable with a facelift alone.

The incisions for the forehead lift are made at the top of the head, generally behind the hairline. The skin above the brows is lifted and redraped over the bone structure, bringing the eyebrows up and smoothing the skin of the forehead. Some trimming of the muscle tissue may take place, with the surgeon carefully avoiding the nerves running throughout the area. The excess skin is removed and sutures close the incision.

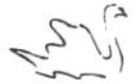

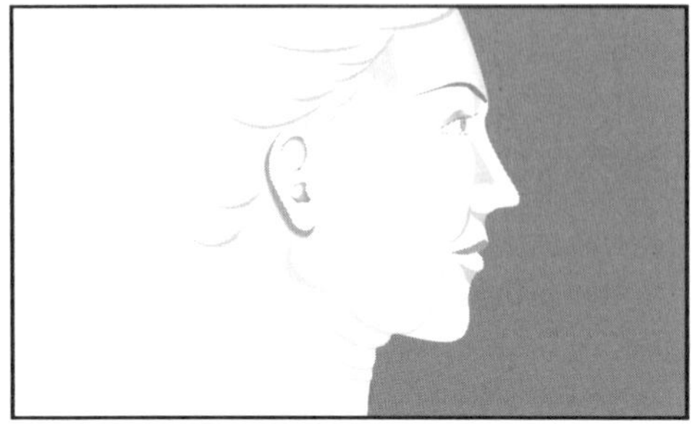

Preoperative facelift patient with excess skin in the face, jowls and neck regions.

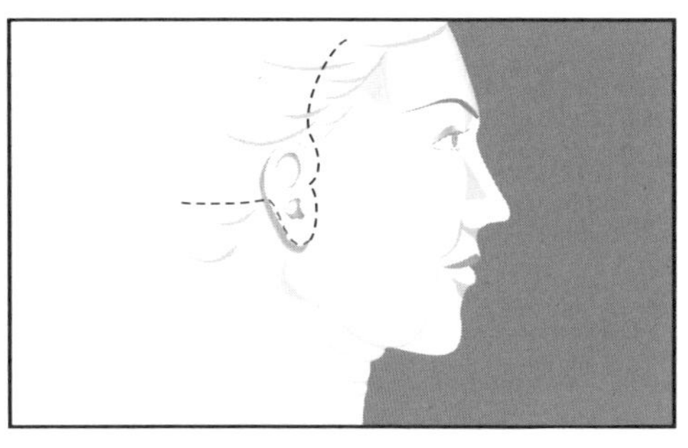

These lines represent the location of incisions commonly made during the facelift procedure: in front of and behind the ears, on the scalp within the hairline and , sometimes, behind the chin. Incisions may vary depending on the technique that your surgeon uses.

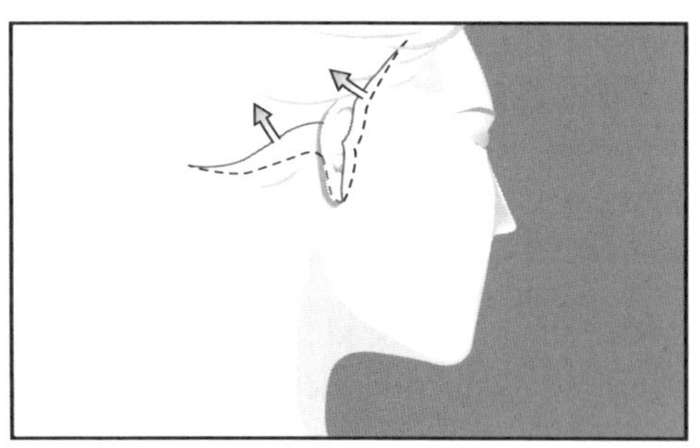

Excess skin is removed and repositioned over the facial contours.

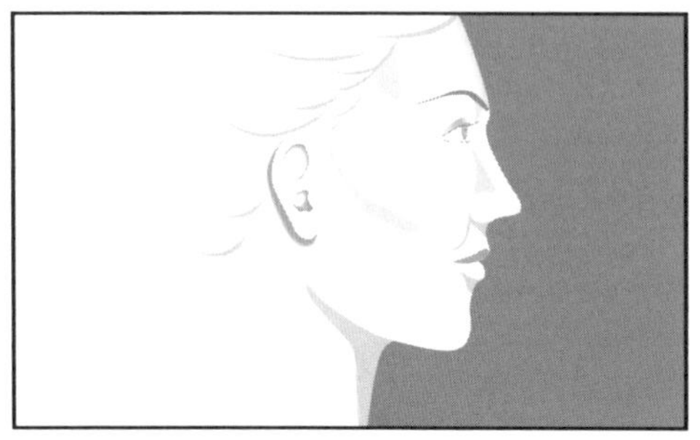

Postoperative facelift patient with a more relaxed, fresher appearance.

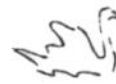

An **eyebrow lift** is a less common procedure recommended for patients who plan a facelift. Men are sometimes steered toward the eyebrow lift rather than the forehead lift. This is generally due to the possibility that, should a gentleman begin to bald, a receding hairline could expose the forehead lift scars made within the hairline.

In the eyebrow lift, a small incision is made in one of two places: slightly above the hair of the brow, or in a natural wrinkle or crease of the forehead. A small section of skin is removed, bringing the brow up and thus restoring the brow to its natural position.

THE POSTOPERATIVE PERIOD

Immediately following the completion of your surgery, you will be monitored to assure that you are recovering well from the anesthesia and are not experiencing any immediate complications from the operation. The doctor and his staff, as well as the anesthesiologist, will maintain this surveillance for an hour or more, until you are fully "out from under" the anesthesia.

If your surgery took place in a hospital, you will be moved from the recovery area to your room within a couple of hours. If your facelift was done on an outpatient basis, you will most likely be moved to a quiet post-surgery area to rest. Some surgeons will recommend that you spend the night after your operation in their care, and may have an over-night facility on the premises. If this is the case, someone on the doctor's staff will stay with you to monitor your condition during the night. This nurse or other care-giver will be keeping an eye on your vital signs as well as looking for signs of hematoma, excess bleeding or swelling. You may also have ice or cold compresses applied to the affected areas throughout the first twenty-four hours.

When the plastic surgeon is ready to release you to go home, he will give you a list of postoperative instructions to follow. For the overall benefit of your health and healing, pay strict attention to these instructions and ask the doctor or his staff about any specific issues or activities on which you are unclear. Some of the items that the doctor will most likely mention are:

- **Medication** - the doctor may prescribe both an antibiotic (to avoid infection) and a mild pain medication to alleviate the discomfort that you may feel in the first few days following surgery. Be certain to take all medication as directed; antibiotics are generally to be taken until all of the pills or capsules are gone. ***Aspirin and aspirin-containing products are to be avoided for up to two weeks following surgery. Ask your doctor.***
- **Pain and discomfort** - expect a feeling of tightness throughout the face and neck. Slight discomfort (the level varying from patient to patient) should be anticipated throughout the facial area, at the incision sites, and at the

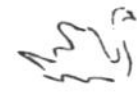

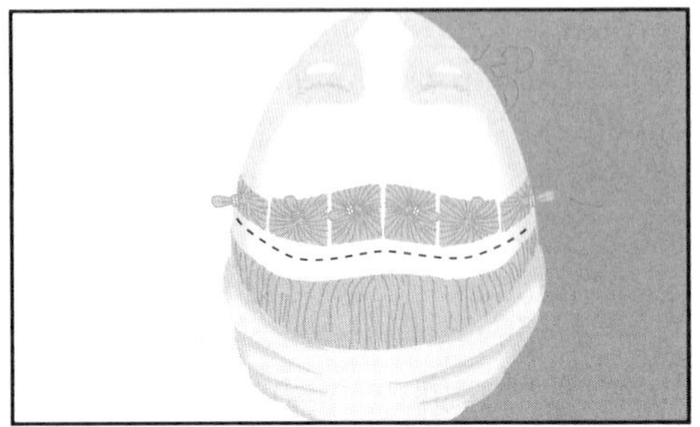

The forehead lift incisions are made behind the hairline and extend horizontally across the scalp.

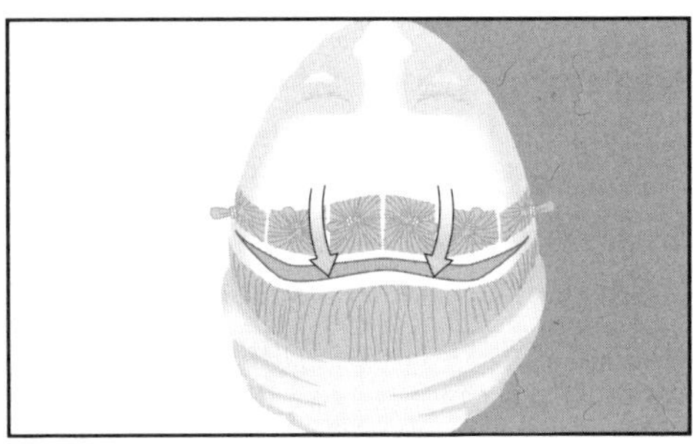

Forehead skin is pulled taut and excess skin is removed. Some surgeons will use different techniques depending on your unique problem areas.

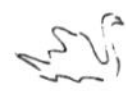

outside of the ears. This should diminish quickly, but don't hesitate to speak with the surgeon should you feel extremely uncomfortable.

- **Swelling** - a considerable amount of swelling in the face and neck almost always presents itself in the first few weeks after the facelift. The doctor will recommend that you **apply iced compresses** on the eyes or other affected regions for the first twenty-four to forty-eight hours following surgery. You should try to **maintain a semi-upright position** as much as possible for the first few days, such as in a recliner chair. If using pillows, **place them behind the shoulders rather than behind the head**, as this may tilt the head forward and put tension on the incisions behind the ear. In bed, try to keep the head at about a **thirty degree angle**. Discuss pillow positioning with your surgeon. In addition, you should **sleep on your back** - try to position yourself to avoid inadvertently rolling onto your side or stomach during the night. You may want to ask your sleep partner to move to another bed for a few nights - an accidental elbow in the wrong place could be very uncomfortable! Lastly, you should probably try to limit your salt intake for a few weeks, since we all know that salt contributes to fluid retention. **NOTIFY YOUR SURGEON IMMEDIATELY IF ANY RAPID OR UNUSUAL SWELLING OCCURS.**
- **Bruising and discoloration** - it is natural for the body to react to the trauma experienced during the facelift by bruising. Your face and neck will go through various stages of bruising, and you may feel as though your entire face is a kaleidoscope. Expect to have many shades of bruising, from black eyes to a nice purple hue to an olive tint, as the healing progresses. It may be several weeks before you are completely bruise-free, and in rare cases, localized discoloration may form as brown spots which can take a few months to heal. You may want to have a heavy make-up and concealers on hand to help mask the bruising when the doctor approves their use.
- **Bleeding** - some bleeding in the first day or so after surgery is common. Most surgeons will install small drains to express most of the bleeding beneath the skin, and will instruct the patient on the care and operation of the drains and reservoir. Drains are usually removed within the first three days after surgery. It is very important to notify the doctor of any unusual bleeding or if a localized area begins to swell rapidly and is painful. This swelling and discomfort could signal bleeding under the skin, or hematoma, and requires the surgeon's attention.
- **Numbness** - is a common condition in the first several weeks after surgery. This is generally seen in localized areas throughout the face, cheeks and neck and is almost always temporary, clearing within several months. In rare cases, nerve damage has occurred during surgery and lack of sensation and/or loss of function in an area will continue permanently.

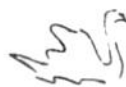

- **Bandages** - the bandaging of the face and neck will vary by surgeon. Some surgeons may leave small surgical tape strips on the incision sites for up to a week.
- **Sutures** - Some of the stitches may be taken out as early as the second or third day after surgery, along with any drains the surgeon implanted. All of the sutures and staples will most likely be out within a week to ten days after the facelift.
- **Scars** - the scars resulting from facelift surgery will go through several phases of healing. The incisions themselves should be healed within a few weeks. For a short period the scars may be very pink, but within a few months the scars should "settle" and become scarcely noticeable, lying within the hairline and the normal creases of the ear.
- **Temporary Postoperative Depression** - a mild case of depression is common in surgical patients, usually occurring within the first postoperative week. Some medications can contribute to the "blues", so let your doctor know what you're taking. It is completely normal to feel a little let down - you have been through a major operation, your activity is restricted, you don't feel up to par, and, quite frankly, you probably don't look so terrific during this period. Don't be unduly alarmed by your negative feelings. They should soon pass, and you will be back to your normal level of activity within a few weeks. Ask your doctor when you can begin walking for exercise, since this may help lift your spirits.
- **Restricting Activity** - In the first few days after surgery your doctor is going to want you to remain as quiet as possible and to rest a great deal. You should have someone with you for the first forty-eight hours after surgery, as you will need help preparing meals, etc. Driving should not be undertaken for the first few days. Talking should be limited, and neck movement should be restricted while the bandages are still in place. No excitement is recommended, and visitors (not that you'll want any!) should be kept to a minimum. For the few days immediately following surgery, you'll want to limit your diet to soft foods and foods that are easily chewed. Bending over at the waist is a no-no: avoid this activity. It will be a day or so before the surgeon approves a full bath or shower and/or washing your hair. Hot rollers, hair dryers and harsh chemicals (such as hair dye or permanent waves) should be avoided for the period specified by your doctor, certainly not within the first couple of weeks. Makeup should only be used when okayed by the doctor, and don't wear earrings until you are fully healed. If you have questions about any specific activity, ask your surgeon. If it's strenuous, if you may become overheated, or if it will put tension on the incision areas he will probably recommend that you wait a week or two.

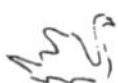

The instructions given to you **by your doctor** should be followed closely. We have mentioned generalities here, and each case is different. As a rule, you should not plan on resuming your normal social activities for about three weeks. Make no mistake about it -you will probably not want a lot of people to see you during the recovery period. No matter how wonderful the ultimate results of your facelift, there will be a couple of weeks in which you want to hide out in the privacy of your own home.

RESULTS

Unfortunately, plastic surgery does not stop the aging process. After a facelift, your face and neck will continue to age at a normal pace, right along with the rest of your body. What a successful facelift *can* do is to reverse or diminish some of the signs of aging that are present at the time of your surgery. In effect, you're "rolling back the clock" five or ten years, appearance-wise. Be advised, though, that the clock doesn't stop ticking.

Most patients feel that they come away from the facelift procedure with a crisper, fresher and smoother appearance. Results can vary to a significant degree from patient to patient, depending, of course, on the condition of the skin and supporting tissue at the time of surgery. **A good facelift is one that is not obvious.**

As a rule, fair skin that tends to be dry usually wrinkles to a greater degree, and the effects of the facelift will not last as long as procedures done on oily, darker skin.

There *are* some actions that the patient can take to prolong the pleasant changes in appearance generated by the facelift:

- If a weight loss is being considered, go on that diet before the facelift. Drastic weight loss contributes to the sagging of facial muscles and skin.
- Try to use a sunscreen **each and every time you sunbathe**. The damaging effects of exposure to the sun have been well documented.
- Avoid facial massage and facial exercises that "stretch" the muscles and skin. As we age, our tissue just doesn't have the ability to bounce back that it used to.
- Try to get into the habit of sleeping on your back. Don't give gravity any help in its constant pull on our anatomy.
- Talk to your plastic surgeon about the skin care products that are most effective against the effects of aging. Preventative medicine is always best.
- Remember, most surgeons will stress that a good facelift is one that is not obvious to strangers

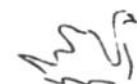

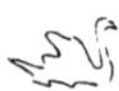

CHAPTER FIVE

NOSE AND CHIN PROCEDURES

"Tis not the lip or eye we beauty call. But the joint force and full result of all"

Alexander Pope
An Essay on Criticism (1711)

In researching this chapter of our book, we conducted a small informal survey amongst our friends and associates. We asked each person, "If you could change one thing about your appearance, other than weight, what would it be?" An astounding seventy-eight percent replied, "My nose." True, this informal survey is certainly not scientific and its results may not reflect the feelings of a nation, but it confirmed something we had thought to be factual in the first place - not many people are really overjoyed with their own nose.

Maybe you inherited Uncle Bernard's nose, with a hump in the middle and oversize nostrils. Or possibly at some point in the past you have taken a blow to the face and sustained a lasting nasal disfigurement from the injury. Perhaps you feel that your nose is too wide, too big, has a hooking appearance, or is bulbous. Some people feel that they can get through life just fine with the nose they have - others dislike this feature to such an extent that they decide to visit a plastic surgeon to discuss **rhinoplasty**, or "nose job".

Nose reshaping is one of the few cosmetic procedures that seem to cross the boundaries of gender. According to data gathered by the ASPRS from its members, over twenty-five percent of the almost seventy thousand nose reshaping procedures performed in 1990 by ASPRS members were done on men. In fact, nose reshaping is the most common cosmetic procedure undertaken by men.

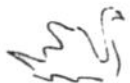

A new nose isn't restricted to the wish list of youngsters, either. While fifty-seven percent of the nose procedures performed in 1990 were done on patients whose ages ranged from nineteen to thirty-four, a full twenty-seven percent of the procedures were undertaken by adults aged thirty-five to fifty. In addition to a life-long dislike of the nose or a nose disfigured through injury, *time* can alter this feature so that it is no longer pleasing to its owner. Gravity can also do its dirty work, pulling the tip down and changing the plane of the nose significantly.

In fact, nose reshaping is the fifth most popular cosmetic surgery procedure performed by members of the ASPRS. The 1990 numbers reflect a twenty-five percent growth over the number of "nose jobs" done by that society in 1981. Many surgeons feel that the breaking down of the stigma associated with having plastic surgery is contributing to the increases. Greater numbers of "nose haters" are taking matters into their own hands, so to speak, and undergoing surgery in order to improve their appearance.

As with all cosmetic procedures, the patient should approach nose reshaping surgery with *improvement*, rather than perfection, as the goal. The surgeon is likely to advise the patient during the consultation process that he will strive for a nose that is in harmony with the rest of the face, both in shape and proportion. Going to the plastic surgeon's office with a picture cut from a magazine of a model's "perfect" nose is fine, so long as you realize that the nose in that picture may not be perfect for your face nor achievable through surgery, given your unique characteristics. Be aware that many plastic surgeons will try to discourage a patient from drastically altering a nose whose shape is a result of ethnic origin. The same rules apply to those noses, as well - the nose should be *in harmony* with the rest of the face. That is not to say that redefining an ethnically shaped nose is out of the question, but rather that the surgeon will probably recommend a subtle rather than drastic change.

There is also another group of nose reshaping patients - those who have a functional or breathing problem. Most commonly, these types of dysfunctions are attributable to a **deviated septum** or other nasal structure defect, where the "breathing space" of the nose is diminished. In these cases, the doctor can repair the breathing dysfunction and combine a certain amount of nose reshaping during the same surgery. Patients with a possible breathing dysfunction should check with their insurance company prior to surgery, since the functional part of procedure may be covered by health insurance.

Because of the influence that the nose has on the aesthetics of the entire face, the surgeon may also recommend a change to the chin. The nose and chin share responsibility for a "balancing act" in regard to the face. Too large a nose with a receding chin is not a look that many patients are happy with, nor is too flat a nose with a prominent chin. There are endless combinations of nose/chin relationships;

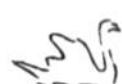

the surgeon will evaluate your unique combination of features during the consultation visit and make recommendations that he feels will give you the results that will please you the most. We will also cover chin procedures in this chapter, due to the frequency with which the two types of procedures are combined into one surgery.

WHO IS A CANDIDATE FOR NOSE RESHAPING?

In general, almost anyone in good health and with the right motivation and expectation of results (see Chapters One and Two) is a good candidate for nose surgery. During your evaluation, the cosmetic surgeon will be examining your nose and its relationship to the rest of your face. If you divide your face into three sections, the "ideal" nose falls entirely into the middle third. The *width* of the "ideal" nose, when viewed from the front, should have the outside edge of the nostril in line with the inner corner of the eye. It is with these ideals in mind that the surgeon will determine the amount of reshaping (if any) needed for your nose. Other than structure, two of the primary factors in determining your candidacy for an effective nose reshaping are *age* and *skin texture*.

In regard to the issue of age, plastic surgeons do not generally recommend cosmetic surgery on the nose of a patient prior to their mid-teen years. This is due to the maturity of the face and bone structure. Most males have a "mature" face in the age range from about eighteen years old; girls, sixteen or older. If a severe disfigurement exists the surgeon will be more apt to bend this criteria, of course. Older patients have no problem with structural maturity, of course. The surgeon's concern with reshaping the nose in a patient of advanced age would be the elasticity of the skin (will it redrape properly over the new nasal structure?) and assuring that the bones of the nose are not too brittle to work with during surgery. In any case, a person should proceed with the consultation process and let the surgeon determine the candidacy of the specific patient.

Skin texture is a primary factor due to the inherent "draping" characteristics of different types of skin. Thicker skin is generally less receptive to the altered bone and cartilage structure, and may not produce results as pleasing as patients with thinner, less coarse skin can achieve. Also, the skin at the tip of the nose is generally much coarser than that at the bridge, so the doctor must evaluate how effective the surgery can be in situations where a great deal of reshaping is needed on the nasal tip.

If a functional problem (such as a deviated septum) exists with the nose, the surgeon must also evaluate the corrections that will be necessary to the nasal structure in order to correct the dysfunction.

Your plastic surgeon will, of course, do a full evaluation of your condition at

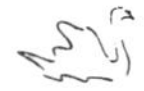

the time of consultation. Some of the things that he or she will be looking at are:

- Your overall health
- Facial Shape
- Age
- Any Nasal Trauma
- Skin Elasticity
- Skin texture and thickness
- Bone and Cartilage Structure
- Hereditary Factors
- Normal Breathing Function
- Shape of Nose Tip

Again, in some cases the surgeon may recommend that the nose reshaping procedure be combined with chin surgery. For this reason we will include a discussion of chin procedures later in this chapter.

RISKS AND COMPLICATIONS

All surgery carries the possibility of complications that are detrimental to the health and well-being of the patient. Commonly, however, perhaps the most troubling complication of nose reshaping is disappointment in the results, which can generally be attributed to the unrealistic expectations of the patient and/or unforeseen variables in postoperative healing. Most surgeons will paint a conservative picture of the results during the consultation process in an attempt to bring the expectations of the patient in line with what is achievable through surgery.

At the time of consultation, your surgeon will discuss with you the most common risks and complications associated with nose reshaping surgery. Some of the issues that he will most likely mention are:

- **Bleeding**: Most common in the first day or two after surgery. Generally appears as a slight discoloration of mucous drainage in bandages beneath the nose. Patient will be provided gauze dressings to be changed as necessary for up to a week. Excessive activity can cause heavier bleeding and should be avoided. Secondary session of bleeding may occur ten to fourteen days after surgery.
- **Bruising**: To be expected for up to three weeks following surgery. Black and blue eyes are not uncommon. Ice compresses can be applied to help alleviate bruising and swelling for the first one to two days after surgery.
- **Swelling**: Heaviest in the first week after surgery, continuing to a noticeable degree up to about six weeks. Some swelling will persist for up to a year or more, with the full effect of the nose reshaping surgery not fully evident until that time.

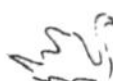

- **Nasal Congestion or dryness**: both are very common;congestion is caused by swollen and irritated mucous membranes. Incisions and coagulated blood in the nose contribute to stuffy feeling. Generally clears within a few weeks, but can persist (in rare cases) for a year or more. Dryness is easily treated with saline spray.
- **Skin Blemishes/Abnormal Pigmentation**: Not common. In some cases, patients experience permanent uneven skin pigmentation (dark spots) or spider veins as a result of surgery. Subsequent treatment (such as chemical peel) may be effective for uneven pigmentation.
- **Infection**: Although very rare, this is always a possibility. Doctor will generally prescribe antibiotics in an effort to avoid infection. Patients should take care to avoid putting any object into the nose that is not specifically approved of by the surgeon. Some surgeons will recommend a treated cotton swab to be used for cleaning the inside of the nostrils during recovery.
- **Breathing Dysfunction**: Some patients experience a change in normal breathing function, similar to stuffy nose or symptoms like those associated with a deviated septum, following rhinoplasty. Most will clear within a few months to a year, some have permanent dysfunction.
- **Irregularities**: A small percentage of patients can be left with slight indentions, ridges or other irregularities after nose reshaping surgery. Most irregularities are correctable with secondary surgery.
- **Disappointment:** Perhaps the most common risk of rhinoplasty. Patients must be aware that a skilled surgeon will avoid "over operating" on a nose, that is, changing a nose so that it no longer works in harmony with the rest of the face. A percentage of patients end up scheduling additional surgery to further change the nose, unhappy with the conservative approach that the surgeon took with the initial procedure. Patients should exercise restraint and give the first rhinoplasty at least a full year to "settle" before scheduling subsequent nose reshaping.

These are some of the risks and complications that rhinoplasty patients should be aware of prior to consenting to surgery. This list is not complete, in that other complications may occur that we have not mentioned. There is no such thing as "minor" surgery, and patients should educate themselves and make an informed decision, fully aware of possible risks and complications, before undergoing any surgical procedure. Discuss this subject in detail with your surgeon and his staff.

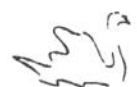

COST

The expense associated with your nose reshaping procedure can vary to a substantial degree, depending on what type of surgical facility your plastic surgeon chooses to utilize. If your doctor feels that a hospital stay is necessary for your operation, the overall cost of your procedure will be greater than one that is done on an outpatient basis. Some nose reshaping patients can anticipate a hospital stay ranging from one to three days, depending on their unique situation and the recommendation of the surgeon. *Most* nose procedures are being done on an outpatient basis; only fourteen percent of the nose reshaping surger-ies performed by members of the ASPRS in 1990 were done on an inpatient basis.

The anesthesia of choice for your operation will be a factor in your final cost, as well. General anesthesia is almost always administered by a physician anesthesiologist whose fees are separate and above those charged by the surgeon, while local anesthesia with sedation is frequently administered by a nurse or the surgeon.

The *average* surgeon's fees for nose reshaping procedures done in 1990 by members of the American Society of Plastic and Reconstructive Surgeons were:

LOW	AVERAGE	HIGH
$300	**$2590**	**$6000**

You should be aware that surgeon's fees will differ throughout geographic regions of the country. In general, prices are somewhat higher on the east and west coasts, with the least expensive procedures available in the interior regions of the United States. These are generalities and should not be used to measure the fees charged by your surgeon. Make certain that you discuss *all* of the costs involved for your procedure, including anesthesiologist fees, post-operative care, etc. prior to surgery day.

As with most cosmetic procedures, the cost of nose reshaping done strictly for cosmetic reasons is not usually covered by health insurance. If performed to correct a nasal or breathing dysfunction, part or all of the surgery costs may be covered. Check with your insurance carrier prior to scheduling surgery. Most surgeons will want at least a partial payment of their fees prior to surgery. If your operation is to be performed in a hospital, separate arrangements may be necessary to cover those expenses.

If you are to have chin surgery, be certain to get the total cost for all procedures to be done during your surgery. The costs for chin reshaping can run from $1000 to $3000, if done as a separate operation. Discuss this in detail with your surgeon and his staff.

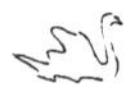

PREOPERATIVE INSTRUCTIONS

At the time that you schedule your procedure, either the doctor or someone on his staff will review with you some instructions that you should follow in the days or weeks immediately prior to your surgery, as well as for the day that your procedure is to be done. Some of the more common cautions that most surgeons will include are:

- Do not take any medication containing aspirin for up to two weeks prior to surgery (can cause excessive bleeding). In addition, your surgeon may recommend that you discontinue use of some hormone medications and certain vitamin supplements - *check with your doctor*!
- The surgeon may advise that the patient take additional Vitamin C for a few days prior to surgery, and some surgeons may prescribe an antibiotic to be taken for a specified number of days before surgery
- Stop cigarette smoking (affects healing).
- No alcoholic beverages up to forty-eight hours prior to surgery.
- Nothing to eat or drink after midnight the night before surgery.
- Arrange for someone to drive you to and from the surgical center, as well as a responsible adult to be with you for twenty-four to forty-eight hours following your release.

Some tips to consider that may not be mentioned: stock up on soft foods and foods that are easily chewed - you're not going to be up to rigorous chewing for the first few days after surgery. Also, purchase a good *liquid* oral hygiene product. Brushing your teeth may be a little uncomfortable for a few days. Lastly, have a supply of "quiet" activities on hand to keep you busy for the first few days of your recovery. Reading, listening to music, television, needle work, etc. will help you pass the time.

ANESTHESIA

A high percentage of plastic surgeons will recommend that the nose reshaping surgery be done at an outpatient surgical center or in his own surgical facility, under either heavy sedation and local anesthetics or under general anesthesia. If sedation and local anesthetics are used, they may be administered by a nurse or the doctor himself. Even though you will not be unconscious under this heavy sedation, you will most likely be sedated to a degree that you "nap" throughout the procedure. To remove the possibility of physical discomfort in the area of the incision, a local anesthetic will be administered after the sedation has had time to

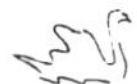

make you relaxed. The prick of the needle and subsequent burning or stinging sensation as the local anesthetic is injected may be slightly uncomfortable, but will soon pass.

If you and your surgeon agree that general anesthesia is the best choice for your operation, odds are that a physician anesthesiologist's services will be required. With general anesthesia, you will be unconscious throughout the procedure. Usually, the anesthesiologist will "put you under" after a mild sedation has been administered to relax you, and the doctor has completed his preoperative preparations.

Be certain to read Chapter Two. Both local and general anesthetics have risks and complications that you should be aware of prior to surgery. While complications attributable to anesthesia range from the mild and common to the severe and rare, you owe it to yourself to be knowledgeable about the subject.

THE NOSE RESHAPING PROCEDURE

Many plastic surgeons consider rhinoplasty (nose reshaping) to be the most difficult cosmetic procedure to master. A certain amount of artistry and anatomical architecture is involved in reshaping the nose, and the physician must perform a balancing act between what is appropriate for the patient's overall appearance and what the patient may think is desireable. The surgeon must strive for the results that will most please the patient while avoiding an "over-operated" look, where the nose no longer fits in with the entire facial package.

Remember that the surgeon is not restoring a feature to its prior appearance, such as in a facelift or blepharoplasty. The nose reshaping procedure will produce a feature that the patient has never actually seen or touched, but rather which has probably been the subject of a life-long fantasy. The patient has most likely spent a number of years visualizing his or her "new nose", and has great expectations for the results of the surgery. In addition, this "new nose" is very difficult to predict with 100 percent accuracy: the postoperative swelling may take up to a year to fully subside, so that the patient must play a waiting game of lengthy duration before being able to appreciate the permanent results.

The good news is that most rhinoplasty patients are more than pleased with the final outcome of their nose reshaping surgery. A small percentage elect to undergo a second nose procedure at a later date to "fine tune" the appearance of the nose, but, by far, most patients are satisfied with the results of the first surgery.

Virtually all of the surgeon's work done during the nose reshaping procedure takes place *inside* the nose, so that little or no visible scarring is present. The exact procedure will differ from patient to patient, depending on what work needs to be

done to that particular nose. Bear in mind that, usually, no skin will be removed during this surgery, so the changes must be done in a manner that will allow the skin to redrape properly over the new nasal structure. This is one of the reasons that skin texture and elasticity play such an important role in determining whether a patient is a good candidate for cosmetic nose surgery.

When you arrive at the outpatient surgical center, hospital or the doctor's own surgical suite, you'll most likely have a brief interview with the nurse and/or anesthesiologist. In addition to taking your blood pressure, etc., you will be asked several questions regarding your medical history and overall health. Some of these questions may be identical to those that you answered at the time of consultation, but the anesthesiologist wants to assure that all the bases are covered and that no surprises await him or the surgeon in the operating room.

After your preoperative examination, the anesthesiologist or nurse will probably give you a mild sedative to help you relax prior to surgery. Next, your face will receive a thorough cleansing using an antibacterial soap. After your sedative has had time to relax you, you will probably have an IV inserted into your arm or wrist. This is used to regulate fluids to be given to you during surgery, as well as providing a means for the speedy injection of any medication necessary during the operation. In addition, the nurse or anesthesiologist will probably have taped some wires to you, in order to monitor your vital signs during surgery.

It is at this point that you may see the surgeon for the first time since your arrival, as he begins marking his "road map" on your nose. These marks, made with a surgical pen (don't worry, it washes off!), will act as a guide for the changes that doctor intends to make during surgery.

If you are to be under general anesthesia for your operation, the mask will probably be fitted over your face now. In a matter of seconds, you will be in a deep unconscious state and will not awaken until after the surgeon has completed his work. If you are to be given local anesthetics with heavy sedatives, the drug will probably be administered now, through the IV tube in your arm. You will begin to drift off, and will most likely be in a deep "nap" when the local anesthetics are injected.

With the anesthesia out of the way, the surgeon is ready to begin his work. The format of your surgery will be determined by the changes to be made to your nose. Below we will give you a general idea of how some of the more common modifications are accomplished. These are in no specific order - your surgeon will work on your nose in a manner that he has determined to be best.

As we have mentioned, the incisions for nose reshaping surgery are made *inside* the nose. The surgeon separates the skin from the underlying bone and cartilage.

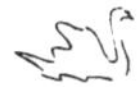

If your nose has a "hump" or "bump" on the bridge, it will be removed utilizing either a rough file called a *rasp* or a small chisel. The surgeon will trim the upper cartilage and/or bone to smooth out the lateral contour of the nose. The doctor will also use this method to trim a nose of height, if that is a problem.

If your nose is too wide at the bridge, the surgeon may weaken the bone and push it together, creating a narrower structure for the skin to drape over.

Reshaping the tip of the nose is tricky business. If the tip needs to be more up-turned, the surgeon will probably shorten the septum (cartilage running down the middle of your nose) and trim the lower and upper cartilage. If the nose has a "hooked" appearance, the surgeon may remove part of the lower cartilage. If your nose is too wide at the tip, the surgeon may trim cartilage and revise the size of your nostrils.

Reducing the size of the nostril is usually the only part of the procedure that may require incisions to be made outside the nose. In the case of oversized nostrils, the surgeon will remove a small section of skin from each nostril at the base. Sutures will bring the tissue together, and each nostril is reduced in size. The incisions usually lie in the natural fold of the nose, and thus are scarcely noticeable, if they can be detected at all.

Once all the trimming and cutting are completed, the doctor will close the incisions made inside your nose. Most surgeons will use a suture material that decomposes, so that the stitches will disintegrate or "fall out" on their own. Only those incisions made at the base of the nostrils will be closed using sutures that will need to be removed, usually in two to four days after surgery.

The dressings applied to your nose will depend on what took place during your surgery. Some procedures require that *packing* be applied inside the nose. This packing will generally remain in place from two to seven days after surgery.

The dressings applied to the outside of the nose may include a *splint* (generally a hard plastic or plaster of paris shield that fits over the top of the nose) as well as surgical tape and gauze. These dressings are used to keep the newly repositioned bone and cartilage in place, as well as to help the skin adjust to the new underlying structure. Most external dressings will be removed within six or seven days following your operation.

After the surgeon has completed his work, you'll probably be moved to a quiet postoperative area where the nurse and/or anesthesiologist will monitor your initial recovery period. In almost all cases, the doctor will release you to go home within a few hours.

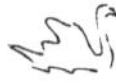

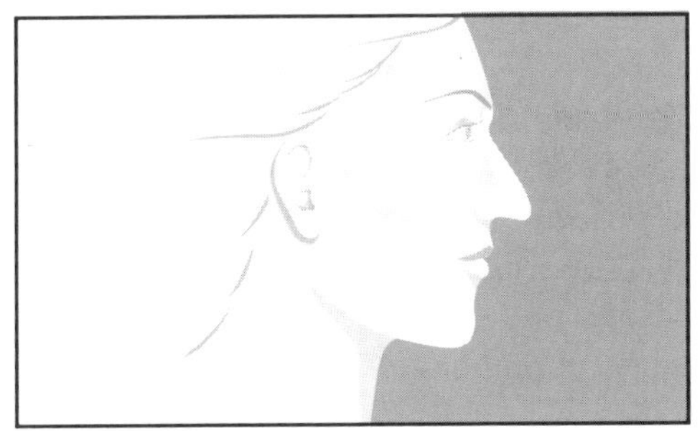

Preoperative nose reshaping patient with a large nasal hump, thick nasal tip and long nasal profile.

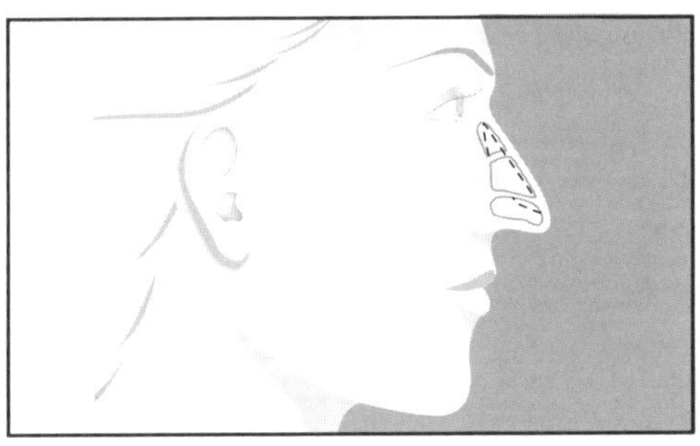

Incisions are commonly made inside the nostrils to allow the surgeon to remove excess bone, cartilage and tissue.

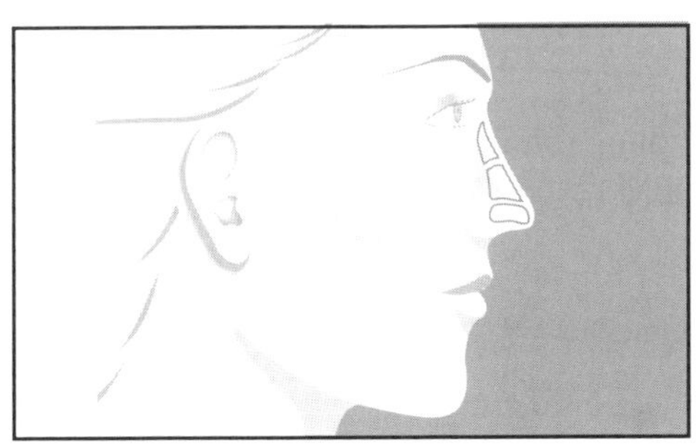

After the removal and reshaping of bone, cartilage and tissue, the skin of the nose will adapt to the new nasal contour.

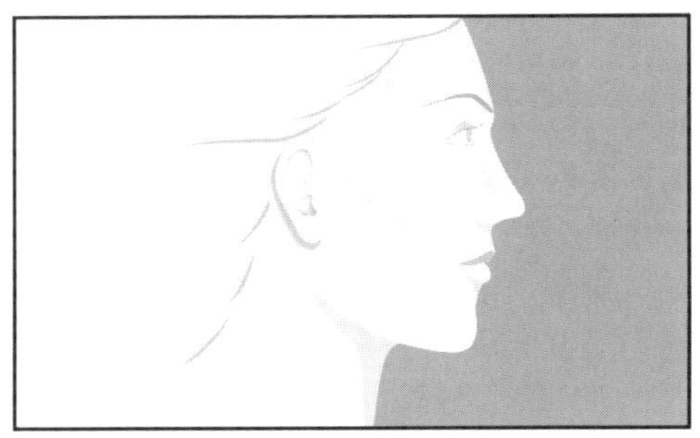

Postoperative nose reshaping patient with a reduced nasal hump, thinner nasal tip and shorter nasal profile.

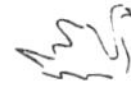

THE POSTOPERATIVE PERIOD

In the hours immediately following surgery, don't feel surprised if you feel as though you've gone a few rounds with a heavyweight boxing champion. You may feel a certain amount of pain, for which the doctor will prescribe medication to be taken for up to a few days after surgery. You will probably have some mucous discharge from your nose into your bandages, and it may include a small amount of blood. You will have to breathe through your mouth for a couple of days until the packing is removed.

You will probably experience a certain amount of bruising and discoloration extending up into the eye area. Swelling is expected, and your nose will probably feel large, tight and stuffy for at least a week or more. Depending on how you feel, you may be ready to return to work in as little as a week or so.

Some of the postoperative instructions and observations that the surgeon will give you:

- **Bleeding** should subside within a few days after surgery, if activity is kept to a minimum during the initial recovery period.
- **Bruising and discoloration** is usually pretty heavy for the first day or two, and black and blue eyes are not uncommon. It may take as long as two weeks for all of the discoloration to disappear.
- **Swelling** will be heaviest in the first few days after surgery, and you will still be considerably swollen when your dressings are removed after six or seven days. Most of the swelling will subside within three to four weeks, with about eighty percent of the swelling diminished by the sixth week after surgery. Remember that it can take up to a full year or more for all of the swelling to completely disappear.
- **Elevate your head** with a couple of pillows when resting or sleeping. This will help alleviate swelling and prevent excessive bleeding. Your bed partner may want to sleep elsewhere for a night or two, since a wayward elbow during the night could cause some serious discomfort.
- If low-grade fever is experienced after surgery **DO NOT TAKE ASPIRIN**. Ask your doctor about any medication to be taken during recovery.
- Eat soft, easily chewed foods for a couple of days.
- **Ice compresses** should be applied to the eyes for a day or two, being careful not to get the bandages wet. Cold water washclothes may be more comfortable than ice bags.
- The surgeon will give you gauze to change the dressing beneath your nose as is necessary. Don't be surprised if this is needed fairly frequently during

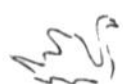

the first day or so after your operation. Any excessive bleeding should be reported to the doctor.

- **DO NOT BLOW YOUR NOSE** for at least a week or two. This could cause bleeding. Try not to put anything in your nose for that period unless instructed to do so by your surgeon, even though you may feel as if you need to clean your nostrils.
- Try to keep quiet for the first day or two after surgery; conversation should be limited; excitement and excesive activity should be avoided. If you have to sneeze, try to do it through your mouth.
- You will probably be given an antibiotic to be taken after your surgery. Remember, most antibiotics are to be taken until all of the prescribed pills are gone.
- **Stuffy nose** is a common complaint of rhinoplasty patients, usually lasting a couple of weeks or more. Your doctor will probably recommend medication.

Most nose reshaping patients can resume normal activity, within reason, after about a month. Strenuous activity such as contact sports and swimming underwater or scuba diving should be avoided for a couple of months. Sun exposure should be avoided as much as possible. Avoid letting eyeglasses or sunglasses rest directly on the nose for a month or so. You may want to utilize your splint or some surgical tape to support the glasses for this period.

These are general instructions only; you should follow the guidelines given to you by your cosmetic surgeon. If you have any questions on specific activities or concerns, contact your surgeon.

RESULTS

Recovery from nose reshaping surgery takes patience. As we have stated before, the full impact of your new nose will not be apparent for as long as a year, since a small degree of swelling may persist for that period. When the dressings are removed after about a week, you may have considerable swelling. Try not to judge the final product by what you see in the mirror at this early juncture - your new nose will emerge slowly over the coming weeks and months, like a butterfly making its way from a cocoon.

Your nose will continue to age at a normal rate, will age contributing to the drooping of the nose tip. The changes made to your nasal structure during surgery are permanent.

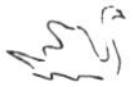

CHIN AUGMENTATION

As we have discussed earlier in this chapter, the nose and chin share a unique relationship. These two features help create a balance in the face, and a drastic change to the nose may further highlight an aesthetic problem with the chin. The most common chin procedure is **augmentation**, used to correct a chin that recedes. Some people refer to this as a "weak" chin. Be aware that the procedure that we discuss here is one that is undertaken for purely cosmetic reasons. Surgery to correct a jaw/chin dysfunction is generally much more involved than an augmentation done merely to enhance appearance.

It is common for plastic surgeons to suggest that the chin procedure be combined with the nose reshaping surgery. When the two procedures are done in tandem, the results can be astounding. Your plastic surgeon will discuss chin surgery with you at the time of consultation, if he feels that the procedure may be needed to accomplish the overall change in appearance that you are looking for.

In chin augmentation, one of two methods are most commonly used. Both methods involve making a small incision beneath the chin, in the natural crease between the chin and lower lip, or inside the mouth. Some surgeons prefer to then cut and *slide forward* the "chin bone", increasing the projection of the chin. The bone is wired into position and the incisions closed.

The other option open to the surgeon is the use of a *silicone implant* to augment the chin. In using the implant, the surgeon does not alter the structure of the bone itself, but rather places a small silicone implant beneath the skin, fitted to the front of the existing bone. This additional mass brings the chin forward. The implant is then sutured in place and the incisions closed.

You should be aware that the silicone used in these implants is currently under scrutiny by the FDA, and is being studied for possible contribution to health risks. Some experts believe that silicone may play a factor in such problems as autoimmune diseases, which include lupus and some forms of arthritis. Discuss the current information available on silicone with your surgeon and make an informed decision based on the facts at hand.

The chin will be taped after surgery, and the surgeon will highly recommend that the patient maintain a soft diet for at least four or five days after surgery. Some discomfort is expected with the chin procedure, and the doctor will probably prescribe a mild medication for pain.

Discuss the chin procedure in detail with your cosmetic surgeon. Make certain to review all risks and possible complications, including the safety of implant devices, before making your decision to undergo the procedure.

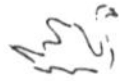

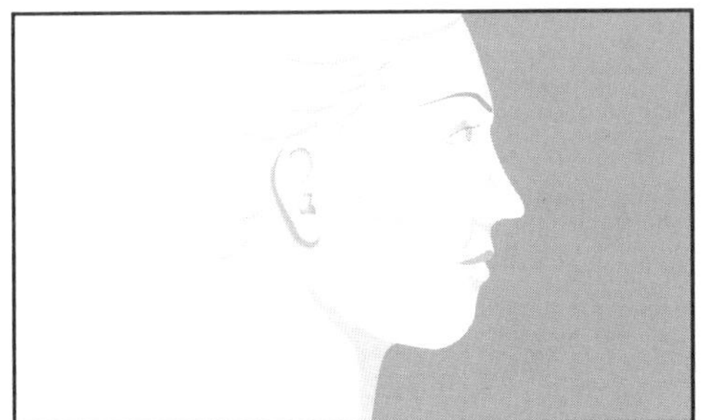

Preoperative chin augmentation patient with a receding chin that is out of balance with other facial structures.

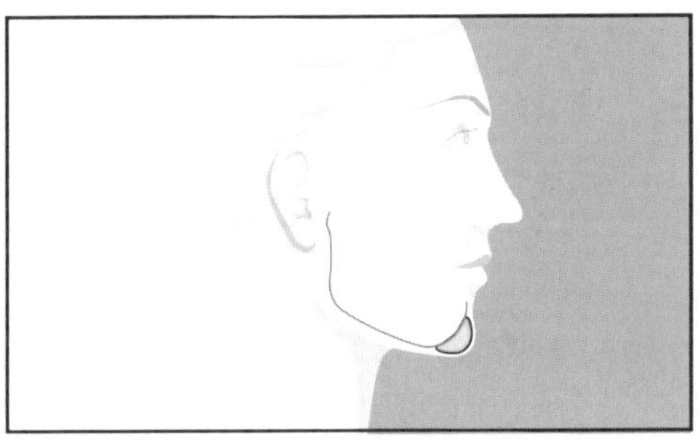

Incisions are made under the chin or inside the lower lip area. The implant is inserted to bring the chin projection forward. Other procedures can be performed without implants that may achieve similar results.

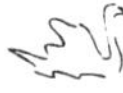

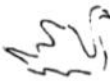

CHAPTER SIX

BREAST REDUCTION

"Beauty is nothing other than the promise of happiness"

Stendhal
On Love (1822)

From the time a young girl enters puberty and throughout the following years of her life, a part of her sense of femininity is associated with her breasts. Some of this deep-seeded relationship between a woman and her breasts is surely due to the biological function that they serve - to nurse her young. Another facet to this complex relationship, however, is based on the attention that breasts receive as a sensually prominent part of the female anatomy. Young teenage boys have been known to spend no small amount of time speculating on which of their female classmates have developed breasts, and in what quantity. For whatever psychological reason, from that point on some men seem to spend the rest of their lives fascinated by the subject. In magazines, television and everyday life, women are constantly bombarded with society's image of the "ideal" woman. It's no surprise, then, that women quickly become painfully aware of any perceived inadequacy in their breasts, whether they be too small, too large or not of the perfect shape.

In cases where Mother Nature has gotten a little overzealous in the bustline department, a woman can feel as though her breasts are out of proportion to her body size and stature. In addition to the aesthetic factors, over-sized breasts can contribute to a number of physical discomforts: back and shoulder pain, poor posture, permanent spinal problems, discomfort when trying to exercise and skin irritation from bra straps are common complaints of women who have breasts that

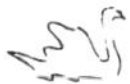

are very large. For some women the condition is so unwanted, uncomfortable and unpleasant that they choose to seek medical assistance in correcting their problem.

According to data gather by the ASPRS from its members, over 40,000 breast reduction (or *reduction mammoplasty*) procedures were performed in 1990 by that group. The vast majority (46%) of these patients were between the ages of 19 and 34, with a small percentage (6%) seeking a plastic surgeon's help before age 18.

The female breast is, technically, the mammary gland. It is made up primarily of fatty and glandular tissue, nerves, milk glands, blood and blood vessels. Running from the breast to the nipple are milk ducts that are used, of course, when a mother breast-feeds her child. Around the nipple is an area of darker skin called the *areola*. This entire breast mass sits atop a chest muscle, which in turn stretches across the ribs. Breast reduction surgery serves to make the breast smaller by the removal of some of the redundant fat and breast tissue, with the appropriate amount of skin cut away and the nipple repositioned to create a aesthetically pleasing shape.

WHO IS A CANDIDATE FOR BREAST REDUCTION?

In theory, almost any woman in good health and with the right motivation for and expectations of results (see Chapters One and Two) is a good candidate for breast reduction surgery. As a rule, though, the patient should be of an age that the breasts have reached their mature size. Young girls who are extremely troubled by oversized breasts or who are experiencing physical discomfort may be considered prior to maturity, but with a special advisement that the procedure may have to be repeated if the breasts are still too large when development is complete.

Young women who are planning to have children should consider the fact that it is highly likely that the reduction procedure will damage the milk ducts to such an extent that breast feeding is impossible. If this is an important issue to the potential mother, the reduction surgery should be delayed until all childbearing has taken place.

New mothers who have recently breast fed babies may want to delay a reduction procedure, since breasts have been known to decrease in size following pregnancy and lactation. Your surgeon should be advised if any infection developed during breast feeding, since this could effect postoperative healing.

Lastly, obese or severely overweight women should attempt to lose weight *before* undergoing breast reduction surgery. In addition to problems associated with anesthesia and surgery, healing is generally considerably slower in obese patients. And since drastic weight loss contributes to sagging breasts, why wait until **after** you have your new look to lose weight and thus risk diminishing your results?

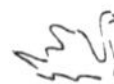

Your plastic surgeon will, of course, do a full evaluation of your condition at the time of consultation. Some of the things that he or she will be looking at are:

- Your overall health
- Body Weight
- Muscle tone
- Skin Elasticity
- Skin type and coloring
- Amount of fat and tissue to be removed
- Body Structure and Build
- Age

Women who are comfortable with the size of their breasts but have marked sagging are not candidates for breast reduction surgery, but should consider the uplift procedure instead. We will discuss the uplift surgery in Chapter Eight.

A note to remember - breast reduction *does leave visible scars*. If this is going to bother you more than the current size and/or shape of your breasts, you should reconsider having the surgery. Note the location of the incision sites in our drawings on this procedure. Include this scarring in your decision-making process.

A final word of advise - *make sure you and your surgeon agree on the approximate post-operative breast size. Serious disappointment and dismay can result if you expected postoperative breasts that are drastically different in size than what your surgeon has in mind.*

ANESTHESIA

Most plastic surgeons will recommend that the breast reduction procedure be done in the hospital, since it is considered major surgery. According to the ASPRS, 81% of the reduction procedures performed in 1990 were done on an *inpatient* basis. General anesthesia is most routinely used for this surgery, and is administered by a physician anesthesiologist.

Under general anesthesia, you will be in a deep unconscious state throughout the surgery. In addition, a mild sedative may be given prior to surgery to help calm your nerves and help you to relax. General anesthesia carries with it some risks and complications that should be considered prior to consenting to surgery, ranging from the common to extremely rare. Some of these complications are: nausea, chipped teeth, sore throat, fever, allergic reaction, even heart attack or death. *Be sure to read Chapter Two!*

COST

The expense associated with your breast reduction procedure can vary to a substantial degree, depending on what type of surgical facility your plastic surgeon chooses to utilize, how long of a hospital stay is necessary for your operation, and the normal fees charged by surgeons in your geographical area. Some reduction

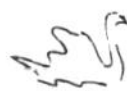

patients can anticipate a hospital stay ranging from two to five days, depending on their unique situation and the recommendation of the surgeon.

The anesthesia of choice for your operation will most likely be general anesthesia, administered by a physician anesthesiologist. This medical specialist's fees are separate and above those charged by the surgeon. Be certain to get the anesthesiologist's fees in advance to determine the total cost of your surgery, as well as that for the hospital.

The *average* surgeon's fees for breast reduction procedures done in 1990 by members of the American Society of Plastic and Reconstructive Surgeons were:

LOW	AVERAGE	HIGH
$1500	**$4040**	**$8000**

Again, you should be aware that surgeon's fees will differ throughout geographical regions of the country. In general, prices are somewhat higher on the east and west coasts, with the least expensive fees available in the interior regions of the United States. These are generalities and should not be used to measure the fees charged by your surgeon. Make certain that you discuss *all* of the costs involved for your procedure prior to surgery day, including anesthesiologist fees, post-operative care, hospital costs, etc.

Unlike most cosmetic procedures, the cost of many breast reduction procedures are covered by health insurance. If persistent and severe back, shoulder and neck pain is present in your situation, you may ask your surgeon to help in determining if part or all of the costs can be covered by your health insurance. In any case, most surgeons will want payment of their fees prior to surgery. Find out in advance what arrangements need to be made with the hospital and anesthesiologist. Some hospitals have a very lenient repayment schedule, others do not. Discuss this in detail with the surgeon's staff, the anesthesiologist's office and the hospital.

RISKS AND COMPLICATIONS

Aside from the risks associated with the general anesthesia (review Chapter Two), there are several possible risks, complications and draw-backs that should be considered when making the decision to undergo breast reduction surgery:

- **Bleeding** - any surgery that involves areas containing blood vessels and veins includes the risk of excessive bleeding.
- **Hematoma** - is, basically, bleeding beneath the skin. If the bleeding does not subside fairly quickly, the surgeon may have to reoperate to close the

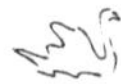

offending blood vessels. Small hematomas can sometimes be taken care of without second surgery by expressing the blood with a syringe.

- **Scarring** - as we mentioned earlier in the chapter, the scars from breast reduction surgery are generally visible after healing. Usually, the surgeon will cut around the *areola, vertically down the breast from the areola to the breast fold, and beneath the breast above the fold.* Some patients heal very well and have only faint scars after six months or so, while other patients develop wide, bright pink and/or raised scars. Post-surgical treatments are sometimes effective on the scars, such as steroid treatment and/or scar revision surgery. These post-surgical treatments are not always 100 percent effective, and the patient can experience permanent, prominent scarring. Be aware also that the postoperative breast can feel "lumpy" until the deep scars soften.
- **Numbness** - can be experienced in both the nipple and the breast itself. Most patients experience some degree of numbness, especially in the nipple, that can last up to six months. In rare cases, feeling and sexual response in the nipple can take years to return, or could be permanent.
- **Infection** - the risk of infection always exists in surgery. Although the surgeon will prescribe antibiotics in an effort to prevent infection, it does occur in rare cases.
- **Abnormal pigmentation** - primarily in the areola; it is sometimes seen in cases of patients who do not heal well. The area around the nipple can be left with small localized areas of darker pigmentation.
- **Pain** - is to be expected in the first two or three days after surgery. Pain medication will almost definitely be needed, and will be administered in the hospital. You will probably receive a prescription for a milder pain medication for your initial recovery period at home, up to a week or so.
- **Inability to breast feed** - a large percentage of reduction patients will not be able to breast feed, since some or all of the milk ducts going to the nipple may be severed during surgery.
- **Nipple or skin loss** - will be of major concern to your surgeon, and a situation that he will be working diligently to avoid. Fortunately, it is not a common occurence. This occurs when the blood circulation to skin and/or nipple is impaired. Smoking can be a contributing factor to both skin and nipple loss. Be certain to discuss this with your surgeon.
- **Assymetry of breasts** - is also another primary concern to your surgeon. This condition is when the breasts are noticably different from one another, either in size or shape. Your surgeon will make his preoperative markings extremely carefully, striving for uniformity in the postoperative breasts.

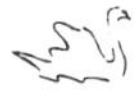

- **Changes in the nipple** - such as lack of protusion or inversion commonly occurs in this type of surgery. In this situation the nipple will lie flat on the breast or may even recess somewhat. There are some minor post-operative procedures that can help rectify an inverted or flat nipple.

These are only some of the risks and complications that should be considered when making the decision to undergo breast reduction surgery. You should discuss this subject in detail with your surgeon and his staff, and be fully aware of the risks and possible complications prior to signing your consent form.

PREOPERATIVE INSTRUCTIONS

At the time that you schedule your procedure, either the doctor or someone on his staff will review with you some instructions that you should follow in the days or weeks immediately prior to your surgery, as well as for the day that your procedure is to be done. Some of the more common concerns that most surgeons will include are:

- Do not take any medication containing aspirin for up to two weeks prior to surgery (can cause excessive bleeding). In addition, your surgeon may recommend that you discontinue use of some hormone medications, birth control pills and certain vitamin supplements - *check with your doctor*!
- The surgeon may advise that the patient take additional Vitamin C for a few days prior to surgery, and some surgeons may prescribe an antibiotic to be taken for a specified number of days before surgery.
- Stop cigarette smoking (may affect healing).
- No alcoholic beverages up to forty-eight hours prior to surgery.
- Nothing to eat or drink after midnight the night before surgery.
- Arrange for someone to drive you to and from the hospital, as well as a responsible adult to be with you for the twenty-four hours following your release from the doctor's care.

Be aware that some surgeons will recommend a pre-surgical mammogram to assure the overall health of the breast tissue. Don't be alarmed, this is an excellent idea and will help assure your continued good health.

Finally, have a supply of "quiet" activities on hand to keep you busy for the first week of your recovery. Reading, television, needle work, etc. will help you pass the time. Try to avoid excitement and visitors for the first few days. Be certain that you understand all of the instructions given to you; call your surgeon's office if you are at all confused.

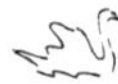

THE BREAST REDUCTION PROCEDURE

Depending on the hospital and your surgeon, you could be admitted either the night before your surgery is scheduled, or just a couple of hours or so prior to the operation. Immediately before surgery you may be given a mild sedative to relax you, then have an IV placed in your arm or wrist. This IV is used to administer fluids and medication before, during and after surgery, and thus will stay in place until well after the operation.

After you are relaxed and prepped for surgery, you'll be wheeled into the operating room. Cardiac monitors will be hooked up (probably high on your chest and back) and another sedative will be administered through your IV. Before surgery, and possibly before your sedative is administered, the surgeon will make his surgical "roadmap" on your chest and breasts. He may have you in a sitting position or standing up. These markings will be made with a surgical pen (don't worry, it washes off!) and will guide the doctor during the operation. One area of particular concern will be the intended new location of your nipple. The surgeon will generally strive for the accepted "ideal" location, which is midway between your shoulder and elbow, at about the same level as the underlying breast fold. The general anesthesia will soon be started and you will lose consciousness.

Working on one breast at a time, the surgeon will operate within a format which he or she is most comfortable. Basically, though, this is pretty much what will go on:

1. The surgeon will remove the skin of a wide key-hole shaped area above the current location of the nipple. The rounded top part of this area is where the nipple will be placed during surgery.
2. Leaving the nipple attached to the breast and thus preserving the nerves and blood vessels, the surgeon will cut *around* the areola and into the lower breast.
3. The redundant fatty and/or breast tissue and excess skin will be removed from the breast, probably in small amounts at a time, with the surgeon judging the size of the revised breast as he operates.
4. When all of the necessary tissue has been removed the nipple will be sutured into place and the remaining incisions will be closed.
5. The surgeon or nurse will cleanse you and then may apply bandages over your breasts. Some surgeons will also apply an "ace" bandage over the gauze, or put the patient in a surgical vest, which resembles an oversized elastic bra.

Bear in mind that in the cases of extremely large breasts (or in procedures involving elderly women) when a great deal of tissue is to be removed and the nipple will be drastically repositioned, the surgeon may have to remove the nipple

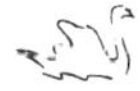

and areola completely and suture them into their new position. This is referred to as a **nipple graft**.

Throughout the surgery the doctor will be using a *cauterizer* to seal blood vessels. You'll not feel this, and it is absolutely necessary to control bleeding. The surgery will usually take between two and four hours, depending on the amount of tissue to be removed, whether or not the nipple can be moved or if it will have to be grafted, and the amount of bleeding experienced during surgery.

After the general anesthesia is discontinued, the anesthesiologist will monitor your immediate postoperative condition in a recovery area. Once he and the surgeon consider you able, you will be moved to your hospital room where you will recover for at least a day, possibly more, before being released to go home.

POSTOPERATIVE RECOVERY

During your recovery period in the hospital, you will have the drains removed that the surgeon placed within your breasts to express any bleeding. Within two or three days after surgery some of the heavy bandages may be removed, to be replaced with a strong supporting bra without underwires. Expect to experience some pain in the first few days, and to continue to feel uncomfortable for up to two or three weeks. Pain medication is generally given by injection in the hospital, then by prescription medication at home. You should also plan on sleeping on your back for the first couple of weeks, and while wearing your special support bra.

The stitches around your areola will be taken out in the doctor's office at around one week after surgery. At your next weekly visit, the surgeon will remove most of the remaining superficial stitches. The remaining sutures will generally be removed sometime between the second and third week after surgery. Removal of all stitches can be a little uncomfortable, but is over quickly. In addition, there are some deep internal stitches that will dissolve on their own. In very small number of patients these degradable stitches don't break down properly and must be removed by the surgeon.

If you have a job that does not involve strenuous activity, the doctor may indicate that it's okay for you to return to work after about two weeks. All activity should be restricted within that first two to three weeks after surgery, since good healing will play a large part in how well your scars will look later. Heavy activity and sports should be delayed for four to six weeks after surgery, or until your surgeon says it's okay. The doctor may recommend that you not have sex for at least three weeks, and no breast manipulation for as much as six weeks.

Expect some bruising for the first week to ten days after surgery, gradually turning to a yellowish discoloration with two weeks. This should disappear completely within a month or so, as should the majority of the swelling. Some

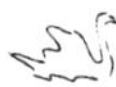

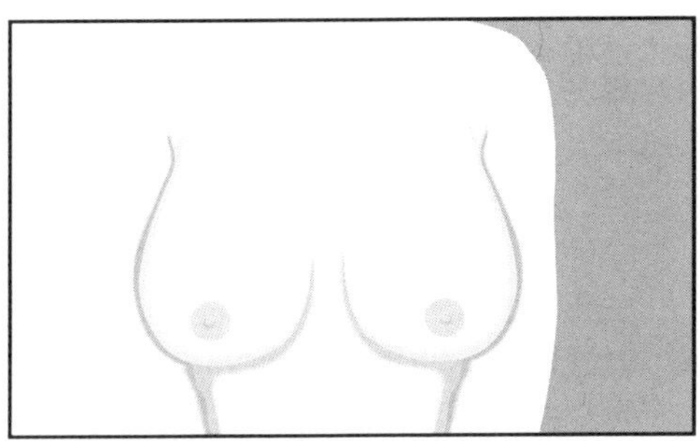

Preoperative breast reduction patient with large, heavy and sagging breasts.

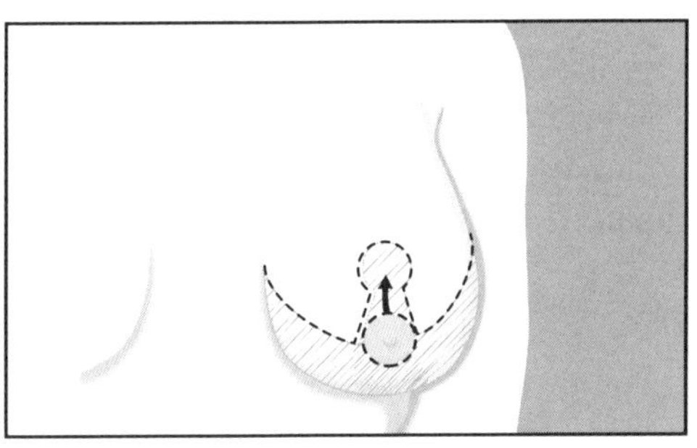

The skin within the dotted lines, in a wide key-hole shaped area, is removed to allow repositioning of the nipple. Excess breast and fatty tissue is removed to reduce the size of the breast.

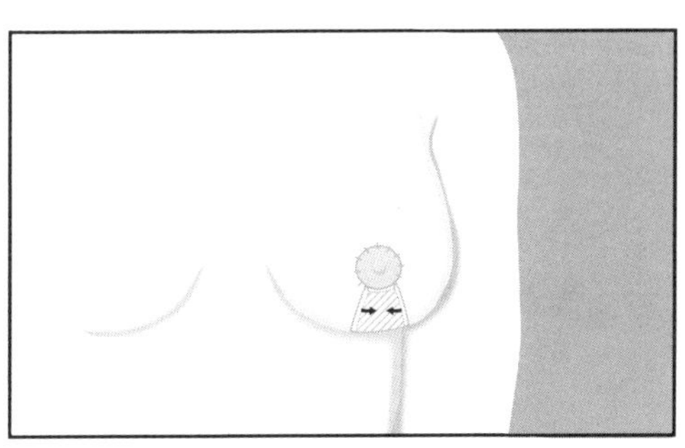

The nipple is sutured into its new position and the incisions are closed.

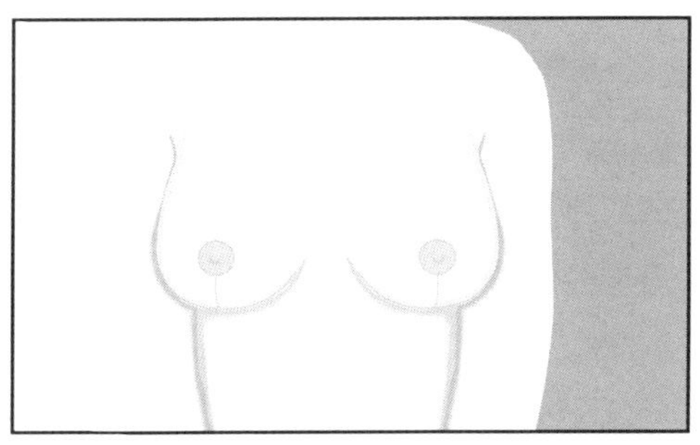

Postoperative reduction patient with smaller, uplifted breasts. Scars are around the areola, vertically down the breast from areola to breast fold, and horizontally above the fold.

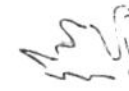

small degree of swelling may persist for months, with the breast "settling" into its new shape and size within three or four months. It may take up to a full year before the final result of the reduction is evident and the scars soften.

RESULTS

The breast tissue, fat and skin that is removed during surgery will not grow back. Watch your weight, though, because *new fat* can still increase the size of your breasts, as may birth control pills, pregnancy, hormone medications and continued breast development due to your age.

Like the rest of your body, the effects of gravity will continue their work and begin to pull the breast downward. And just like everyone else, you may experience some sagging of the breasts as you age. In general, most breast reduction patients are absolutely delighted with their new physique. Be aware of a possible post-operative depression, though, and be prepared to deal with a sense of loss in regard to size of your breasts.

While the vast majority of breast reduction patients are extremely satisfied with their postoperative breasts, some patients may feel less feminine for a short time after surgery, even though they despised the size of their breasts before the operation. Talk to your surgeon should you encounter these negative feelings, and get him to show you your "before" pictures again. If your decision was well thought-out before hand, and if you had realistic expectations of your results before the procedure, your negative feelings should soon pass.

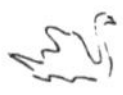

CHAPTER SEVEN

BREAST ENLARGEMENT SURGERY

"Know, first, who you are, and then adorn yourself accordingly"

Epictetus
Discourses (2*nd c.*)
3.1, *tr. Thomas* W. *Higginson*

Throughout the centuries, women who were unhappy with the size of their breasts had little choice but to try and disguise the problem. Flat-chested women, struggling to fit into society's concept of the perfect female form, resigned themselves to stuffing brassieres with everything from cotton balls to bobby socks to facial tissues. For most of our history (except for a few short years in the sixties and early seventies) *voluptuous* has been the fashion, with the old standard of "36-24-36" providing women with a concrete (but pretty much unattainable) goal.

Science has tried to help us out along the way. In the 1950's, the medical community thought that they had developed the very thing to help women who felt that nature had been particularly stingy in the breast-size department. Some physicians injected liquid silicone into breast tissue, increasing breast size *and*, unfortunately, causing extremely serious medical problems.

Back to the drawing board they went, and within the next decade had come up with **silicone implants**. This time, rather than injecting the liquid silicone directly into breast tissue, the substance was in gel form and was enveloped in a silicone rubber pouch. The silicone gel was soft and pliable within its enclosure, and felt very similar to human breast tissue in texture. By surgically placing the implant beneath the patient's own breast, the size of the breast was increased to

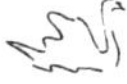

create a physique more to the patient's liking. Word spread fast, and soon the breast enlargement surgery or **breast augmentation**, was the solution that many women had been waiting for to an age-old problem.

In the years since their development in the 1960's, silicone gel implants have undergone a few changes. The implant walls and silicone gel on newer models are much thicker, for example. Prior to a 1991 FDA investigation, they were the most commonly used device for breast augmentation, even though other types of implants have been developed in recent years. Generally, implants have the same outer silicone-rubber pouch; the *contents* of the pouch or the texture of the outer surface of the implant is what differs from type to type.

One device, called the **inflatable** or **saline** implant, is placed in the body *before* its contents are added. Once the surgeon has the device in place, it will be filled with a sterile saline (salt water) solution. The amount of saline solution put into the implant will depend on the amount of breast enlargement desired - the less solution, the smaller the implant. Should the implant leak or rupture, the saline solution is merely absorbed into the system, since it is similar in composition to the body's natural fluids. The down side to this type of implant is that if it does leak or rupture, the implant loses volume quickly (within a few hours) and the breast rapidly decreases in size. Result: more surgery to replace the deflated implant. Underfilled inflatable implants can also "slosh" inside the breast, like the water in a balloon.

Another of the enlargement devices is a hybrid of the gel and saline implants- the **double-lumen** implant contains an envelope of silicone gel lying within an outer pouch of saline solution. The benefit of this type of implant is that it allows the surgeon to adjust the size of the device once it is in place, and, should a rupture or leak occur, the amount of deflation is relatively slight.

The last two types of implants differ from the others in the types of ***texture*** in their outer coating. One of the most common complications of breast augmentation is called **"capsular contracture",** which results in the breasts becoming overly firm with an unnatural feel. In a nutshell, this condition is the body's reaction to the foreign object, the implant. The textured implants were developed in an effort to reduce the degree of capsular contracture. The newest textured device is simply a variation of the standard silicone gel implant, but with a scored or rough outer skin to the pouch.

The other different type of textured implant, developed in the early 1980's, was an implant that had a coating of polyurethane foam. This so called "fuzzy" implant was thought to prevent capsular contracture in a large number of patients, and became very popular in the period immediately following their release. All was not to be rosy with the "fuzzy" implants, however. Within the past couple of years, a controversy has erupted over the safety of the polyurethane coating of these

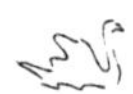

devices. Scientists know that the polyurethane slowly degrades inside the body, and can break down into 2-toluene diamine (TDA), a substance that may have caused cancer in laboratory animals. In response to the findings the manufacturers halted worldwide distribution of the polyurethane coated devices and removed them from the market in 1991.

In January 1992, the FDA asked for a moratorium on the use of *silicone gel* implants. This action came from an increasing concern as to the safety of silicone implants, primarily with the possible negative side effects of silicone released into the body by way of a ruptured device, or through the seepage of silicone gel through the implant wall. Since the FDA has never formally approved silicone implants, the moratorium was called to allow time to study the devices and to address the safety concerns expressed by both members of the medical community and consumer groups. The focus of concern is the effects of silicone gel released into the body from ruptured, leaking or seeping implants. The saline-filled implants were not included in the initial moratorium, but most experts feel that even these devices will ***not*** be spared the FDA scrutiny.

You may be wondering how a device so widely used has never been formally approved by the FDA. When a 1976 law was passed regulating medical devices, silicone implants had already been on the market for over a decade and were "grandfathered" into a category of "assumed to be safe" devices. This allowed the implants to bypass the approval process, and it was not until 1982 that the FDA reclassified silicone implants as needing further research. In early 1991, the FDA notified implant manufacturers that they had three months to produce evidence that the devices were safe. The moratorium on the use of silicone gel implants called for by the FDA in January 1992 was a result of what the FDA felt was insufficient information presented from implant manufacturers as to the safety of their products.

As of the printing of this book, that voluntary moratorium is still in effect. In February 1992 a panel of experts recommended to the FDA that silicone gel implants remain available to patients needing reconstructive surgery (such as mastectomy patients) and, to a very limited number of cosmetic surgery patients. The FDA is to evaluate this recommendation and make a decision on the issue in the not so distant future.

The benefits of breast enlargement are obvious - a woman concerned about the size of her breasts to such a degree that she considers surgery to correct the problem may experience a much improved self-image following the procedure. It is very difficult to get away from that picture of the "ideal" female body, and some women may feel that they want to use any means available to improve their physique. Other women, such as models and actresses may feel that they ***must*** enlarge their breasts for career reasons.

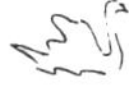

It is extremely important that any woman considering breast augmentation surgery investigate the issues surrounding breast implant devices. By all means, discuss the various options available to prospective breast enlargement patients with your surgeon at the time of consultation. Use the resources available to make an informed decision regarding silicone implants, as well as becoming aware of the risks and complications of breast augmentation surgery. Two sources that you may want to consult in your decision-making process are: The FDA breast implant hotline, 1-800-532-4440; and the American Society of Plastic and Reconstructive Surgeons hotline, 1-800-333-8835.

WHO IS A CANDIDATE FOR BREAST AUGMENTATION?

In general, almost anyone in good health and with the right motivation and expectations of results (see Chapters One and Two) is a viable candidate for breast augmentation. Two of the more important factors in determining whether a patient will enjoy favorable results from an augmentation are *skin elasticity and physical build.*

Your plastic surgeon will, of course, do a full evaluation of your condition at the time of consultation. Some of the things that he or she will be looking at are:

- Your overall health
- Current breast size
- Muscle tone
- Skin elasticity & amount of sagging
- Desired breast size
- Body Build

The surgeon will discuss your expectations as to the size of the enlarged breast to assure that your mental picture of the results of the procedure are as accurate as possible. Very few surgeons will agree to implants that would be much too large for the patient's body build.

RISKS AND COMPLICATIONS

Aside from the risks associated with the anesthesia (review Chapter Two), there are several possible risks, complications and draw-backs that should be considered when making the decision to undergo breast augmentation surgery:

- **Bleeding** - any surgery that involves areas containing blood vessels and veins includes the risk of excessive bleeding. Be certain to discuss the symptoms of excessive postoperative bleeding with your doctor.
- **Hematoma** - is, basically, bleeding beneath the skin. If the bleeding does not subside fairly quickly, the surgeon may have to reoperate to close the

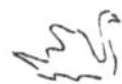

offending blood vessels. Small hematomas can sometimes be taken care of by removing the blood with a syringe, but secondary surgery can sometimes not be avoided.

- **Scarring** - The scars from breast augmentation surgery are generally barely visible after healing. Usually, the surgeon will make his incisions in one of three areas: around the *areola, in the armpit, or beneath the breast above the natural fold*. Some patients heal very well and have only faint scars after six months or so, while other patients' scars may take longer to fade. A small number of patients experience widened or brightly colored scars; post-surgical treatments are not always 100 percent effective for scar correction, and the patient can experience permanent visible scarring.
- **Numbness** - can be experienced in both the nipple and/or the breast itself, depending on where the incisions were made. Most patients experience some degree of numbness, especially in the nipple, that can last up to six months. In rare cases, feeling and sexual response in the nipple can take years to return, or can be permanent.
- **Infection** - the risk of infection always exists in surgery. The surgeon will prescribe antibiotics in an effort to prevent infection, but it does occur in rare cases and can require the removal of the implant. *Very rarely*, a patient may experience toxic shock syndrome.
- **Abnormal pigmentation** - primarily in the areola, is sometimes seen in cases of patients who do not heal well. Again, this would be seen primarily in patients whose incisions were made around the areola. The area around the nipple can be left with small localized areas of darker pigmentation.
- **Pain** - is to be expected in the first two or three days after surgery. You will probably receive a prescription for a mild pain medication for your initial recovery period at home, up to a week or so.
- **Complications from silicone leakage** - are still being studied by the FDA at the time of this printing. Be aware that the implant wall (even on implants filled with the saline solution) are made up, in part, by silicone. Future studies will most likely focus on the outer structure of the device, as well. In addition, some medical experts are expressing strong concern about the possibility of silicone contributing to the development of *autoimmune* diseases such as lupus and some forms of arthritis, although a connection has not be proven as of the date of this printing. Experts are still unsure of the permanent consequences of silicone implants.
- **Capsular Contracture** - is a common complication of breast augmentation surgery. How common is a matter of some debate, with some experts estimating that up to 30 percent of augment patients experience the condi-

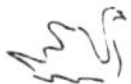

tion to a noticeable degree. Capsular contracture occurs when the body reacts to the foreign body by forming a capsule around the implant. If the fibrous capsule tightens to a sufficient degree around the implant, the breast can become uncomfortably firm and distorted in shape. Treatment for the condition includes a non-surgical technique of the physician squeezing the breast to break up the capsule - often painful for the patient, and with a possibility of rupturing the implant in the process. Other options are to remove or loosen the capsule surgically, and/or replacing the implant. With both techniques, recurrence of the condition is possible.

- **Difficulty in detecting cancer** - in some situations, the placement of the implant or the effect of the implant on normal breast tissue can make it more difficult to detect abnormalities in the breast. A patient should always advise other medical professionals of the implants when seeking care, and should be certain to schedule a mammogram with a radiologist that is trained in the special techniques necessary to properly screen a breast with implants. The "Ecklund" technique is used for this purpose, and may involve additional cost for the mammogram.

These are only some of the risks and complications that should be considered when making the decision to undergo breast augmentation surgery. You should discuss this subject in detail with your surgeon and his staff, and be fully aware of the risks and possible complications prior to signing your consent form.

PREOPERATIVE INSTRUCTIONS

At the time that you schedule your procedure, either the doctor or someone on his staff will review with you some instructions that you should follow in the days or weeks immediately prior to your surgery, as well as for the day that your procedure is to be done. Some of the more common precautions that most surgeons will include are:

- Do not take any medication containing aspirin for up to two weeks prior to surgery (can cause excessive bleeding). In addition, your surgeon may recommend that you discontinue use of some hormone medications, birth control pills and certain vitamin supplements - *check with your doctor*!
- The surgeon may advise that the patient take additional Vitamin C for a few days prior to surgery, and some surgeons may prescribe an antibiotic to be taken for a specified number of days before surgery.
- Stop cigarette smoking - affects healing.
- No alcoholic beverages up to forty-eight hours prior to surgery.
- Nothing to eat or drink after midnight the night before surgery.

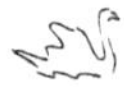

- Arrange for someone to drive you to and from the surgical center, as well as a responsible adult to be with you for the twenty-four hours following your release from the doctor's care.

Be aware that some surgeons will recommend a pre-surgical mammogram to assure the overall health of the breast tissue. This is a good idea to help assure your continued good health.

Finally, have a supply of "quiet" activities on hand to keep you busy for the first week of your recovery. Reading, television, needle work, etc. will help you pass the time. Try to avoid excitement and visitors for the first few days. Be certain that you understand all of the instructions given to you; call your surgeon's office if you are confused about any of the items on his list.

ANESTHESIA

A high percentage of plastic surgeons will recommend that the augment procedure be done at an outpatient surgical center or in his own surgical facility, using either general anesthesia or sedation and local anesthetics.

The procedure will generally last no longer than two to three hours. If sedatives and local anesthesia is used, you will not be unconscious, but you will most likely be sedated to a degree that you "nap" throughout the procedure. To remove the possibility of physical discomfort in the area of the incision, a local anesthetic is administered after the sedation has had time to relax you. The prick of the needle and subsequent burning or stinging sensation as the local anesthetic is injected may be slightly uncomfortable, but will soon pass.

If your surgeon feels that your surgery is best performed with general anesthesia, you will be in a deep unconscious state throughout the procedure, and under the care of an anesthesiologist. Be sure to read Chapter Two to become familiar with the different types of anesthesia, who usually administers each type, and the risks and complications associated with anesthesia.

COST

The expense associated with your breast enlargement procedure can vary to a substantial degree, depending on what type of surgical facility your plastic surgeon chooses to utilize. If your doctor feels that a hospital stay is necessary for your operation, the overall cost of your surgery will be greater than one that is done on an outpatient basis. Some breast enlargement patients can anticipate a hospital stay ranging from one to three days, depending on their unique situation

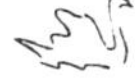

and the recommendation of the surgeon. *Most* augmentation procedures are being done on an outpatient basis; only eighteen percent of the breast augmentation procedures performed by members of the ASPRS in 1990 were done on an inpatient basis.

The anesthesia of choice for your operation will be a factor in your final cost, as well. General anesthesia is almost always administered by a physician anesthesiologist whose fees are separate and above those charged by the surgeon, while local anesthesia with sedation is frequently administered by a nurse or the surgeon himself.

According to data collected by the ASPRS from its members, the ***average*** surgeon's fees for breast augmentation procedures done in 1990 by that group:

LOW	AVERAGE	HIGH
$1000	**$2400**	**$5500**

You should be aware that surgeon's fees will differ throughout geographic regions of the country. In general, prices are somewhat higher on the east and west coasts, with the least expensive procedures available in the interior regions of the United States. These are generalities and should not be used to measure the fees charged by your surgeon. Fees can even differ from city to city within the same state. Make certain that you discuss *all* of the costs involved for your procedure prior to surgery day, including anesthesiologist fees, postoperative care, etc.

As with most cosmetic procedures, the cost of breast enlargement is not usually covered by health insurance. Most surgeons will want payment of their fees prior to surgery. If your operation is to be performed in a hospital, separate arrangements may be necessary to cover those expenses. Discuss this in detail with your surgeon's staff.

THE BREAST ENLARGEMENT PROCEDURE

This procedure is fairly uncomplicated. Once the patient is sufficiently sedated or asleep, the surgeon will make an incision through which he will place the implant beneath the existing breast tissue. The two primary variations in this surgery are *where the implants are placed* and the *location of the incisions*.

The most common locations for the breast augmentation incisions are: near the natural fold of the breast (where breast meets abdomen), around the areola, or, less commonly, in the armpit. The size of the implant to be used is one of the factors that the surgeon will take into consideration when deciding the location of your incisions, as well as your own unique physical characteristics.

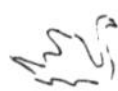

The surgeon has two choices of how to place the implant: either directly behind the breast tissue and in front of the chest muscle; or, if appropriate, behind the breast tissue *and* chest muscle. Some surgeons feel that implants placed behind the chest muscle have less probability of forming capsular contracture (described above, in the Risks and Complications) and it can interfere less with breast self-examination and mammagram. The drawbacks to intramuscular implants are that the recovery time may be slightly longer and may be more painful, it could cause muscular dysfunction, the implant shape can become distorted, and that it is almost always done under general anesthesia. In both types of the procedure, a pocket is formed into which the surgeon places the implant.

Once the device is in place, the surgeon will close the incisions and either place gauze bandages around the breasts and/or put the patient in a surgical (heavy supporting) type bra. The surgery usually takes around two to three hours, and some surgeons may allow the patient to go home within a few hours after recovery from anesthesia. If your procedure was done in a hospital, you may be required to spend the night.

THE POSTOPERATIVE RECOVERY PERIOD

Most surgeons will have you back in their office the day following surgery in order to check your progress and to remove the bandages. Your stitches will be removed within the week, but the surgical or heavy-support bra will probably be required for a couple of weeks.

The majority of augmentation patients will experience some swelling and bruising which will gradually subside within the next two to three weeks. Your surgeon will probably want you to limit your physical activity for the next three to four weeks, but returning to work should not be a problem after the first six or seven days.

Expect to return to the surgeon for intermittent follow-up visits throughout the first year after surgery. The doctor will want to check for complications and to follow your healing progress.

RESULTS

The results of a breast enlargement accomplished using an implant device are, for all intents and purposes, permanent. Unless the implant leaks, ruptures or is removed from the body, the additional volume added to the natural breast size will remain indefinitely.

Patients should bear in mind, however, that this procedure is not insurance against an aging bustline. The breasts will age, for the most part, right along with

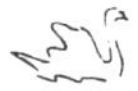

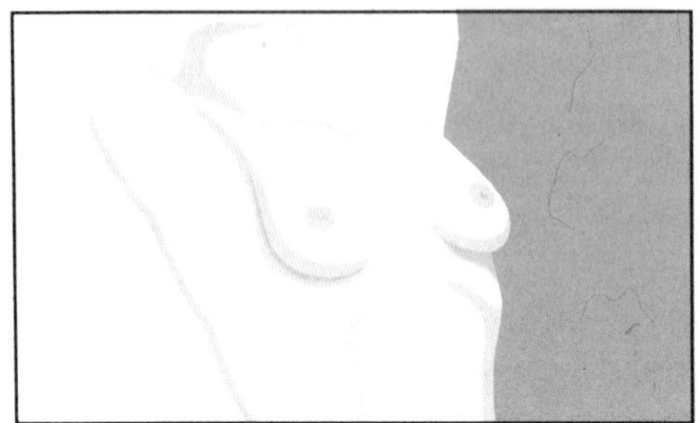

Preoperative enlargement patient with small breasts lacking projection.

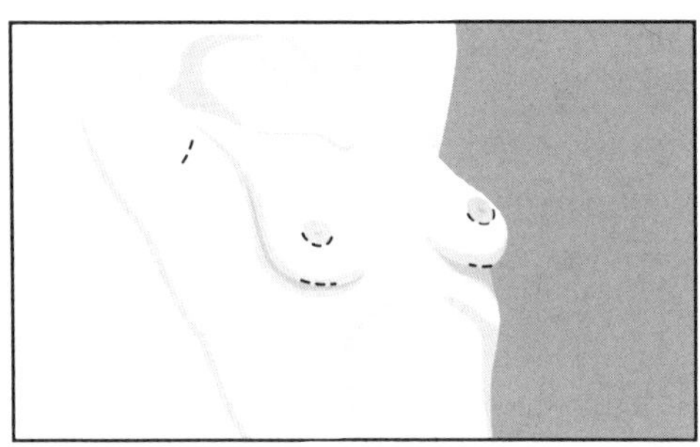

The incisions will either be placed under the breast above the fold, around the lower half of the areola or in the armpit.

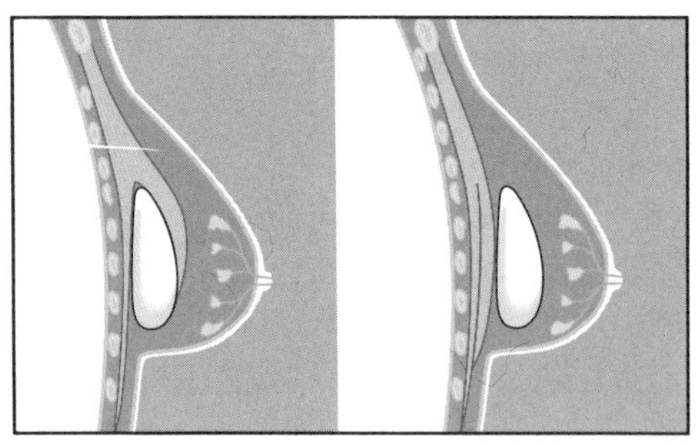

On left, profile of a breast with the implant positioned beneath both the breast tissue and the chest muscle. On right, implant beneath breast tissue only.

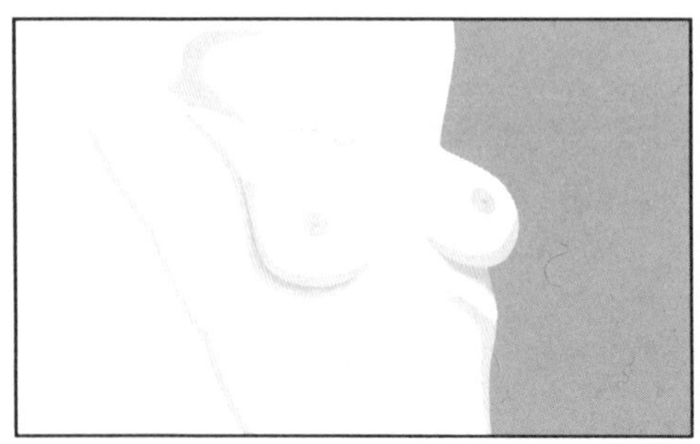

Postoperative breast enlargement patient with fuller breasts.

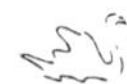

the rest of the body. As skin elasticity decreases, the breasts may begin to sag. In some cases the breast may become disfigured, in that the implant remains in position but the natural breast tissue sags below the area of the implant. Correction would require additional surgery.

As we discussed earlier in the chapter, the benefits of breast enlargement surgery are obvious. In a matter of hours, a woman can have the bustline that she may have been dreaming of for most of her lifetime. In this age of instant gratification and the "easy fix", this can be a tempting solution. Women ***must***, however, take the time to investigate the issues surrounding breast implants and augmentation surgery prior to consenting to the procedure. A number of issues have been raised in the recent past that require the patient to make a well informed, well thought-out decision.

In the best of all worlds, beauty and good health co-exist.

HAVING EXISTING IMPLANTS REMOVED

Based on the best estimates that the silicone implant manufacturers and plastic surgeons can provide, approximately a million women currently have silicone gel implants. About eighty percent of these women decided to undergo breast augmentation surgery for aesthetic reasons (to improve appearance). For these women, the events of recent months have been nerve-wracking at best. What was undertaken to bring about a positive change in their self-image may have turned into a nagging source of apprehension and uneasiness.

Some of these women will, undoubtably, want the implants removed - even if they have not yet experienced any problems attributable to the devices. Be aware that thus far no one has advocated the removal of silicone implants in women not reporting problems. But with all of the publicity, even women who have had no negative experiences with their implants are expressing interest in finding out about their options. Can the implants be safely removed? Will their breasts look like they did before the augmentation procedure?

The first logical step for any woman considering implant removal is a visit to their surgeon. If a woman is unable or unwilling to visit the surgeon who performed the initial augmentation surgery, she should be certain to schedule her consultation with an experienced, qualified surgeon who is familiar with the various breast procedures. Patients should try to bring their surgical records and most recent mammagram with them to the consultation. According to Dr. J. Barry Boyd, a Winter Park (Florida) plastic surgeon, there are several factors that must be taken into account when considering the removal of implants. For simplicity's sake, we will focus only on procedures that will not involve replacing current implants with another type of device:

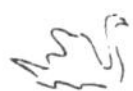

- What type of implant (silicone gel, "fuzzy" implant, etc.) does the patient have? - Coated implants are more likely to have integrated into adjoining tissue, requiring the removal of what your surgeon may refer to as the "capsule", or the hardened tissue that the body forms around the implant.
- Is the capsule thick and does it encompass a large amount of tissue? - Even patients with implants that do not have a "fuzzy" coating can experience bulky, thickened capsules. The surgeon will be more likely to recommend a "capsulectomy" (removal of implant and capsule) if this is the case.
- What is the overall condition of the breast? Will an uplift be needed or desired by the patient? - Under ideal circumstances, the surgeon could merely remove the implant through the original incision sites made during the augmentation surgery. Under these conditions there would be little if any additional scarring. Unfortunately (especially in women who have had implants for an extended period of time) the breast may have lost some of its original volume since the time the implant surgery was performed, either by weight loss, pregnancy, age or other natural causes. These women may be cautioned that the post-operative breast without implants could be likened to a "deflated balloon", and an uplift procedure may be recommended. A note: breast uplift procedures will require additional skin incisions and therefore result in visible scarring.
- What is the psychological outlook of the patient? Has she reconciled herself to the idea of having substantially smaller breasts? - Dr. Boyd indicates that some patients should consider psychological counseling prior to elective implant removal. After all, the augmentation procedure was initially undergone to improve self-image. Is the patient prepared to deal with her feelings after the implant removal?

In addition to the above factors, the surgeon will want to make certain that the patient understands the risks and possible complications of implant removal. As well as all of the risks pertaining to any type of surgical procedure - the possibility of infection, scarring, excessive bleeding and the risks pertaining to anesthesia (to name only a few), the patient should be aware that the possibility exists for skin and/or nipple loss and rupture of the implant in the process of removal. Some of the most common concerns involved in the uplift procedure are discussed in more detail in Chapter Eight. Because of the number of factors to be considered in implant removal surgery the cost of this procedure can vary widely from patient to patient.

During the consultation with the surgeon be certain to get the total cost of this surgery - including the anesthesiologist's fees, hospital expenses, post-operative care, etc. According to Dr. Boyd, "There are also several types of procedures available to exchange ruptured implants for new implants. In addition

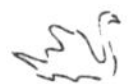

to capsulectomy and implant removal, conversion to a new location (ie: submuscular pocket) and new type (ie: textured saline) are considerations. Ptosis [sagging] correction may also need to be evaluated." Proceed with caution when considering implant removal - be certain that you have given the facts much thought, that you see a qualified surgeon experienced in breast procedures and that you are fully prepared for the condition of your post-operative breasts. Most plastic surgeons will probably not recommend the removal of implants that are intact, but the choice is yours to make.

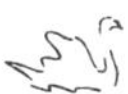

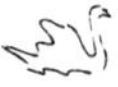

CHAPTER EIGHT

BREAST UPLIFT PROCEDURE

"Time, in the turn-over of days, works change for better or worse."

Pindar
Odes (*5th c* B.C.) *Isthmia* 3,
tr. Richard Lattimore

As with the rest of our bodies, gravity maintains a constant downward pull on our breasts. This persistent force, when exerted on skin that has begun to lose its elasticity, causes the breast to sag. The nipple may drop from its youthful placement to a position that is below the breast fold (where the bottom of the breast meets the body).

The breast uplift procedure **(or mastopexy)** is very similar to the reduction procedure in the site and types of incisions that are made during surgery, but the uplift procedure should be considered by patients looking to correct only sagging breasts, *not breasts that are too large*. During the uplift procedure, no breast tissue will be removed and the size of the breast generally will not decrease. Only excess skin is cut away and the nipple repositioned to create a better contour and shape.

WHO ARE THE BEST CANDIDATES FOR THE UPLIFT?

In general, almost anyone in good health and with the right motivation for and expectations of results (see Chapters One and Two) is a good candidate for the breast uplift surgery if the condition exists to a level that is correctable by surgery. As a rule, the age of the patient has little impact on the prospects for good results in the uplift procedure so long as the level of skin elasticity is such that the skin will

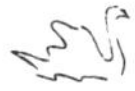

adapt well to the new breast contour. In fact, according to data gathered by the ASPRS from its members, 65% of the breast lift procedures performed in 1990 by that group done on women over the age of 35. Your plastic surgeon will, of course, do a full evaluation of your condition at the time of consultation. Some of the things that he or she will be looking at are:

- Your overall health
- Skin type and coloring
- Skin Elasticity
- Amount of skin to be removed

In some cases, the surgeon may feel that the uplift procedure alone may not accomplish the results that you hope to achieve unless a breast augmentation (enlargement) is done along with the uplift. There is currently much controversy surrounding the silicone implants most commonly used for **breast augmentation**, and the patient *must* take the time and trouble to investigate the pros and cons of augmentation surgery before agreeing to the procedure. Ask the surgeon to give you a realistic idea of what you can expect from the uplift procedure alone (without augmentation) and decide if the results would be satisfactory. If you decide to consider the augmentation surgery, **be certain to read the previous chapter in this book!**

Patients planning to have children or undergo a substantial weight loss in the near future may want to consider postponing the uplift procedure. Both pregnancy and weight loss lend themselves to additional sagging of the breast.

ANESTHESIA

A high percentage of plastic surgeons will recommend that the uplift procedure be done at an outpatient surgical center or in his own surgical facility with mild sedation and local anesthetics administered by a nurse or the doctor himself. In fact, 81% of the breast lift procedures performed by ASPRS in 1990 were done on an outpatient basis. The surgery generally takes no longer than two to three hours. Some surgeons advocate the use of a physician anesthesiologist, even when general anesthesia is not used. This enables the doctor to rely on the anesthesiologist to monitor your vital signs and condition during surgery, freeing the surgeon to concentrate on the work at hand. With sedation, you will not be unconscious during the operation, but you will most likely be sedated to a degree that you "nap" throughout the procedure. To remove the possibility of physical discomfort in the area of the incisions, a local anesthetic will be administered after the sedation has had time to make you relaxed. The prick of the needle and subsequent burning or stinging sensation as the local anesthetic is injected may be slightly uncomfortable, but will soon pass.

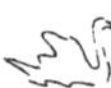

COST

The expense associated with your breast lift procedure can vary to a substantial degree, depending on what type of surgical facility your plastic surgeon chooses to utilize. If your doctor feels that a hospital stay is necessary for your operation, the overall cost of your uplift will be greater than one that is done on an outpatient basis. The anesthesia of choice for your operation will be a factor in your final cost, as well. If general anesthesia is needed for your surgery, or if your surgeon requires the services of a physician anesthesiologist, the cost will be somewhat higher. An anesthesiologist's fees are separate and above those charged by the surgeon.

The **average** surgeon's fees for breast lift procedures done in 1990 by members of the American Society of Plastic and Reconstructive Surgeons were:

LOW	AVERAGE	HIGH
$1000	$2890	$6500

You should be aware that surgeon's fees will differ throughout geographic regions of the country. In general, prices are somewhat higher on the east and west coasts, with the least expensive procedures available in the interior regions of the United States. These are generalities and should not be used to measure the fees charged by your surgeon. Make certain that you discuss *all* of the costs involved for your procedure prior to surgery day, including anesthesiologist fees, postoperative care, etc.

As with most cosmetic procedures, the cost of a breast lift is not usually covered by health insurance. Most surgeons will want payment of their fees prior to surgery. If your operation is to be performed in a hospital, separate arrangements may be necessary to cover those expenses. Discuss this in detail with your surgeon's staff.

RISKS AND COMPLICATIONS

Aside from the risks associated with the anesthesia (review Chapter Two), there are several possible risks, complications and draw-backs that should be considered when making the decision to undergo breast lift surgery:

- **Bleeding** - is not generally a problem, since deep tissues that contain many blood vessels and veins are not usually affected in the uplift procedure.
- **Scarring** - as we mentioned in the previous chapter, the scars from breast reduction surgery are generally visible after healing, and since the incisions

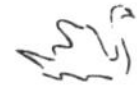

made in the skin for the uplift procedure are very similar to the ones made during a reduction, scarring is a factor to consider. Usually, the surgeon will cut around the *areola, vertically down the breast from the areola to the breast fold, and beneath the breast above the fold.* Some patients heal very well and have only faint scars after six months or so, while other patients develop wide, bright pink and/or raised scars. Post-surgical treatments, such as steroid treatment and/or scar revision surgery, are sometimes effective on the scars. These post-surgical treatments are not always 100% effective, and the patient can experience permanent, prominent scarring.

- **Numbness** - can be experienced in the nipple for a number of months, but rarely is permanent. Although it is rare, feeling and sexual response in the nipple can take years to return, or could be permanent.
- **Infection** - the risk of infection always exists in surgery. The surgeon will prescribe antibiotics in an effort to prevent infection, but it does occur in rare cases.
- **Abnormal pigmentation** - primarily in the areola, is sometimes seen in cases of patients who do not heal well. The area around the nipple can be left with small localized areas of darker pigmentation.
- **Pain** - is to be expected in the first two or three days after surgery. Pain medication may be needed, and a prescription for a mild pain medication will probably be given for your initial recovery period at home.
- **Loss of breast projection** - in some uplifts done without implants to augment the breast tissue the uplifted breast may have very little projection. Discuss this with your surgeon.
- **Nipple or skin loss** - due to lack of circulation and aggrivated by smoking. Although a somewhat rare occurence, subsequent surgery may be necessary to correct nipple and/or skin loss.

These are only some of the risks and complications that should be considered when making the decision to undergo breast uplift surgery. You should discuss this subject in detail with your surgeon and his staff, and be fully aware of the risks and possible complications prior to signing your consent form.

PREOPERATIVE INSTRUCTIONS

At the time that you schedule your procedure, either the doctor or someone on his staff will review with you some instructions that you should follow in the days or weeks immediately prior to your surgery, as well as for the day that your procedure is to be done. Some of the more common items that most surgeons will include are:

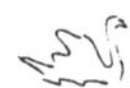

- Do not take any medication containing aspirin for up to two weeks prior to surgery (can cause excessive bleeding). In addition, your surgeon may recommend that you discontinue use of some hormone medications, birth control pills and certain vitamin supplements - *check with your doctor*!
- The surgeon may advise that the patient take additional Vitamin C for a few days prior to surgery, and some surgeons may prescribe an antibiotic to be taken for a specified number of days before surgery.
- Stop cigarette smoking - it affects healing and can contribute to scarring, etc.
- No alcoholic beverages up to forty-eight hours prior to surgery.
- Nothing to eat or drink after midnight the night before surgery.
- Arrange for someone to drive you to and from the surgical center, as well as for a responsible adult to be with you during the twenty-four hours following your release from the doctor's care.

Be aware that some surgeons will recommend a pre-surgical mammogram to assure the overall health of the breast tissue. Don't be alarmed, this is an excellent idea and will help assure your continued good health.

Finally, have a supply of "quiet" activities on hand to keep you busy for the first week of your recovery. Reading, television, needle work, etc. will help you pass the time. Try to avoid excitement and visitors for the first few days. Be certain that you understand all of the instructions given to you; call your surgeon's office if you are confused about any of the items on his list.

THE BREAST LIFT PROCEDURE

Since your procedure will probably be done in an outpatient center or at the surgeon's own office, you will most like be asked to arrive just a couple of hours or so prior to the operation. Immediately before surgery you may be given a mild sedative to relax you, then have an IV placed in your arm or wrist. This IV is used to administer fluids and medication before, during and after surgery.

After you are relaxed and prepped for surgery, you'll be wheeled into the operating room. Cardiac monitors may be hooked up and another sedative will be administered through your IV. You may soon begin to "nap" shortly after this sedative is given, so the surgeon will quickly begin to make his surgical "roadmap" on your chest and breasts while you are still comfortable in a sitting position, if he has not already made his lines and arrows prior to this point. These markings will be made with a surgical pen (don't worry, it washes off!) and will guide the doctor during the operation. One area of particular concern will be the intended new location of your nipple. The surgeon will generally strive for the accepted "ideal"

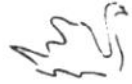

location, which is midway between your shoulder and elbow, at about the same level as the underlying breast fold.

Working on one breast at a time, the surgeon will operate in a format which he or she is most comfortable. Basically, though, this is pretty much what will go on:

1. The surgeon will remove the skin of a wide key-hole shaped area above the current location of the nipple. The rounded top part of this area is where the nipple will be placed during surgery.
2. Leaving the nipple attached to the breast and thus preserving the nerves and blood vessels, the surgeon will cut *around* the areola and trim the excess skin.
3. When all of the necessary skin has been removed and the surgeon is satisfied with the positioning of the nipple, he will suture the nipple into place and close the remaining incisions.
4. The surgeon or nurse will cleanse the torso and apply tape and/or bandages over the breasts. Some surgeons will also apply an "ace" bandage over the gauze, or put the patient in one of their own bras, with gauze protecting the incisions.

Bear in mind that if augmentation is necessary to give you the results that you want from the uplift procedure, additional work will have to be done during the surgery. Be certain to read the chapter on Breast Augmentation.

The uplift surgery will usually take between one and three hours. After the surgeon has completed his work, the IV sedative will be discontinued and you will slowly "come around". Once the surgeon considers you able, you will be moved to a quiet recovery area where you will recover for at least a few hours. After this brief recovery period your chaffeur for the day can drive you home.

POSTOPERATIVE RECOVERY

Expect to be quite sore with some swelling and bruising for the first week or so after your surgery, and plan on getting plenty of rest. Most surgeons will allow their patients to take a shower almost right away, changing the gauze bandages and putting on a clean bra as needed. Some doctors will want you to wear your bra twenty-four hours a day, even while sleeping (on your back! Rolling over on your tummy during sleep could be a little uncomfortable!)

Within five to ten days after surgery, the stitches around your areola will be taken out in the doctor's office. At your next visit the following week, the surgeon may remove the stitches placed underneath the skin. The deepest sutures will be

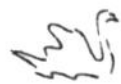

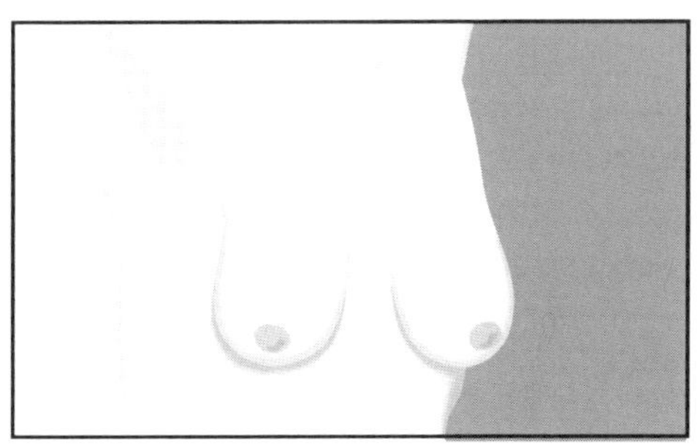

Preoperative uplift patient with sagging, pendulous breasts.

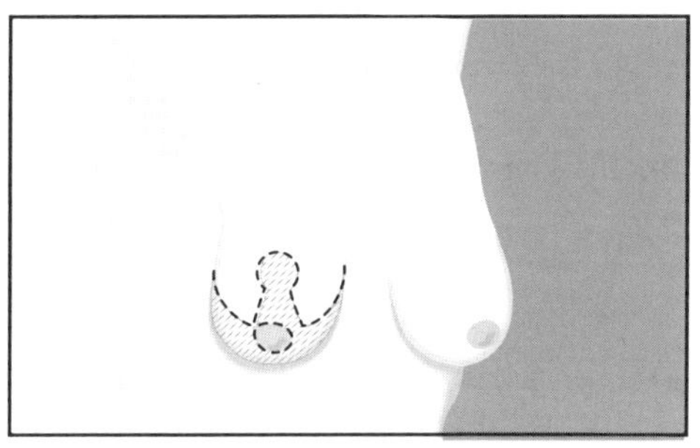

The skin within a wide keyhole shaped area will be removed to allow repositioning of the nipple. Excess skin will be removed.

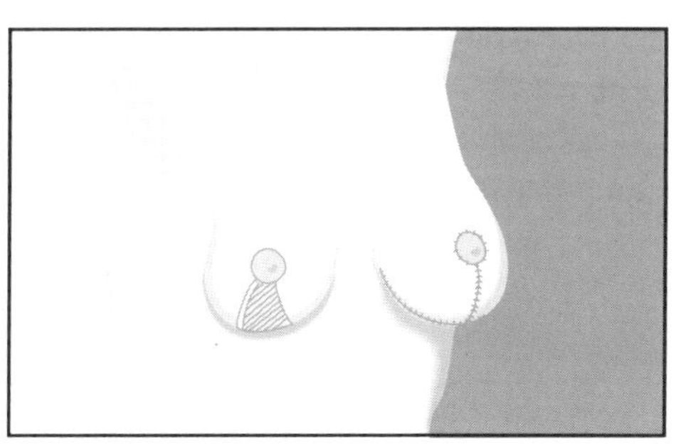

The nipple is sutured into its new position and the incisions are closed.

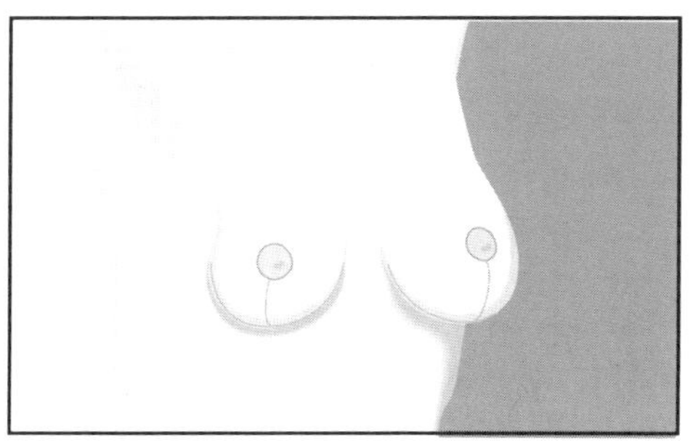

Postoperative breast uplift patient with scars around the areola, vertically from the areola to the breast fold, and horizontally above the fold.

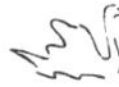

of a "degradable" material, and should dissolve on their own inside your breast. In a small number of patients, these stitches don't dissolve, requiring the surgeon to remove them. Removal of all stitches can be a little uncomfortable, but is usually over quickly.

If you have a job that does not involve strenuous activity, the doctor may indicate that it's okay for you to return to work after about a week. All activity should be restricted within the first two weeks after surgery, since good healing will play a large part in how well your scars will look later. Heavy activity and sports should be delayed for four to six weeks after surgery, or until your surgeon says it's okay. The doctor may recommend that you not have sex for at least two weeks, and no breast manipulation for as much as six weeks.

Plan on wearing your bra almost constantly for a few months - many doctors recommend an athletic type bra that provides alot of support. Remember, the newly reshaped breast needs all the support it can get!

RESULTS

The results of breast lift surgery are not permanent, but you have "rolled back the clock" on the drooping tissues. Be aware that your breasts are not immune from the forces of gravity! As you continue to age, your breasts may begin to droop again over a period of time, but usually not to the degree that they were sagging before surgery. Some tips on keeping your new breasts in their post-surgical shape: Watch your weight, since drastic weight fluctuations can increase your chances of sagging, and wear your bra whenever practical and comfortable. Drooping *can* recur following pregnancy, and/or if you have an inherited tendency to sagging.

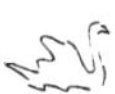

CHAPTER NINE

TUMMY TUCK

"Gracefulness is to the body what understanding is to the mind."

La Roche-Foucauld
Maxims (1665)
tr. Kenneth Pratt

Each year around the beginning of Spring, every woman I know starts to show the unmistakable signs of anxiety and apprehension. Her palms sweat, she suffers from mild depression and she is filled with a sense of dread. She knows that soon, *very soon*, she will be faced with an event more horrifying, more fearsome than any other that will take place during the coming year - *she will be faced with the dreadful day that she must don her bathing suit for the first time since the end of last summer.* It's easy to hide our flaws (even from ourselves) when, for the past four or five months of winter, we've lived in sweat pants and flannel shirts. The horrors faced at this time last year have dimmed in our memory, and we have hope that things aren't as bad as we fear they will be. Maybe those bumps and bulges that made us so self-conscious last year have gone away, miraculously, like the melting of the snow in the March sunshine. Maybe our tummies will lie flat, as in the days of our youth. Or, alas, maybe not.

Most of us, as we age, begin to show a little bulge around the lower tummy. Unfortunately, some women (and men, for that matter) have much more than a little bulge. The skin and muscle, stretched and weakened from pregnancy and/or weight fluctuation or obesity, shows prominent sagging and drooping and "pouches out". Fat accumulates readily in this area, further compounding the problem. In some cases this "apron" of skin can fold over the pubic area, causing skin irritation in the areas beneath the apron. Some women experience a problem with sexual activity due to the excess skin and tissue.

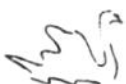

Abdominoplasty, or the *tummy tuck*, is a cosmetic procedure utilized to remove the excess skin and fat in the abdomen. In some cases the underlying muscles are tightened as well. The result is a firmer, flatter tummy. Be aware, though, that prominent scarring occurs with the tummy tuck, and ***it is major surgery***. The tummy tuck is **not** a replacement for a good diet and exercise. Patients who visit a cosmetic surgeon looking for surgery to tighten up a slightly "puffy" tummy that has very little loose skin are likely to be sent to their health spa to work on the abdominal muscles instead.

Most tummy tuck procedures are performed in the hospital under general anesthesia, with the length of stay determined by the extent of the surgery, whether hernias were treated in the operation, and the overall condition of the patient. Some patients whose conditions do not warrant a great deal of work on the abdominal muscle may be treated on an outpatient basis, either at an outpatient surgical center or in the physician's own operating suite. According to data gathered by the ASPRS from its members, of all the tummy tuck procedures performed by that group in 1990, 75 percent were done on an inpatient basis (in the hospital).

WHO IS A GOOD CANDIDATE FOR THE TUMMY TUCK?

In general, almost anyone in good health and with the right motivation and expectations of results (see Chapters One and Two) is a good candidate for a tummy tuck if the condition exists to a level that is correctable by surgery. As a rule, the age or ethnic origin of the patient has little impact on the prospects for good results in abdominoplasty. More important is the general overall health of the patient.

The results of the tummy tuck are permanent, in that the fat and skin removed during the procedure will not "reappear". Subsequent pregnancies or drastic weight fluctuation can weaken and stretch the abdominal muscles again, though, causing a recurrence of the symptoms. Patients considering the tummy tuck should take this into consideration, possibly delaying surgery until a goal weight is achieved and maintained, and/or no more pregnancies are planned.

Your plastic surgeon will, of course, do a full evaluation of your condition at the time of consultation. Some of the things that he or she will be looking at are:

- Your overall health
- Skin elasticity
- Muscle tone
- Health history
- Skin type
- Amount of fat and skin to be removed
- Presence of hernias
- Body Weight and build

In some cases, your surgeon may recommend that the tummy tuck procedure

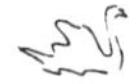

include the use of **liposuction**. Be certain to read the chapter in this book on liposuction if your surgeon indicates that this technique will be used in your surgery.

ANESTHESIA

Most plastic surgeons will recommend that the tummy tuck procedure be done in the hospital, since it is considered major surgery. General anesthesia is most routinely used for this surgery, administered by a physician anesthesiologist. Under general anesthesia, you will be in a deep unconscious state throughout the surgery. In addition, a mild sedative may be given prior to surgery to help calm the nerves and relax the patient. General anesthesia carries with it some risks and complications that should be considered prior to consenting to surgery, ranging from the common to extremely rare. Some of these complications are nausea, chipped teeth, sore throat, fever, allergic reaction, even heart attack or death. Be sure to read Chapter Two!

COST

The expense associated with your tummy tuck can vary to a substantial degree, depending on what type of surgical facility your plastic surgeon chooses to utilize, how long of a hospital stay is necessary for your operation, and the normal fees charged by surgeons in your geographical area. Some abdominoplasty patients can anticipate a hospital stay ranging from two to five days, depending on their unique situation and the recommendation of the surgeon.

The anesthesia of choice for your operation will most likely be general anesthesia, administered by a physician anesthesiologist. This medical specialist's fees are separate and above those charged by the surgeon. Be certain to get the anesthesiologist's fees in advance to determine the total cost of your surgery, as well as that for the hospital. The ***average*** surgeon's fees for tummy tuck procedures done in 1990 by members of the American Society of Plastic and Reconstructive Surgeons were:

LOW	AVERAGE	HIGH
$1200	$3430	$8500

Again, you should be aware that surgeon's fees will differ throughout geographic regions of the country. In general, prices are somewhat higher on the east and west coasts, with the least expensive fees available in the interior regions

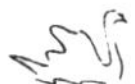

of the United States. These are generalities and should not be used to measure the fees charged by your surgeon. Make certain that you discuss *all* of the costs involved for your procedure prior to surgery day, including anesthesiologist fees, post-operative care, hospital costs, etc.

As with most cosmetic procedures, the cost of a tummy tuck is not usually covered by health insurance if undergone for strictly aesthetic reasons. If persistent and severe skin irritation or other medical conditions are attributable to your condition, you may ask your surgeon to help in determining if part or all of the costs can be covered by your health insurance. In any case, most surgeons will want payment of their fees prior to surgery. Find out in advance what arrangements need to be made with the hospital and anesthesiologist. Some hospitals have a very lenient repayment schedule, others do not. Discuss this in detail with your surgeon's staff, the anesthesiologist's office and the hospital.

RISKS AND COMPLICATIONS

Aside from the risks associated with the general anesthesia (review Chapter Two), there are several possible risks, complications and draw-backs that should be considered when making the decision to undergo the tummy tuck surgery:

- **Bleeding** - any surgery that involves areas containing blood vessels includes the risk of excessive bleeding.
- **Hematoma** - is, basically, bleeding beneath the skin. If the bleeding does not subside fairly quickly, the surgeon may have to reoperate to close the offending blood vessels. Small hematomas can sometimes be taken care of without second surgery by removing the blood with a syringe.
- **Scarring** - as we mentioned earlier in the chapter, the scars from a tummy tuck are generally visible after healing. Usually, the surgeon will make a long incision that runs the width of the torso, just above the pubic area and within the natural creases where the leg meets the body. Some patients heal very well and have narrow scars after six months or so, while other patients develop wide, bright pink and/or raised scars. Post-surgical treatments are sometimes effective on the scars, such as steroid treatment and/or scar revision surgery. These post-surgical treatments are not always effective, and the patient can experience permanent, prominent scarring.
- **Numbness** - can be experienced in the abdominal area, and can last up to six months or more.
- **Infection** - the risk of infection always exists in surgery. The surgeon will prescribe antibiotics in an effort to prevent infection, but it does occur in rare cases.

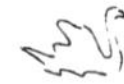

- **Pain** - is to be expected in the first two or three days after surgery. Pain medication will almost definitely be needed, and will be administered in the hospital. You will probably receive a prescription for a milder pain medication for your initial recovery period at home, up to a week or so.
- **Phlebitis** - is the inflammation of a leg vein. Although this is not a common complication, the risk does exist. Phlebitis is sometimes experienced after surgery and/or after periods of extended bed rest. It can be dangerous, since a clot can move throughout the circulatory system and disrupt the normal function of vital organs, such as the lungs.
- **Reposition of the navel** - while not really a complication, occasionally a few patients are not pleased with the new "belly button" placement. Just realize that your navel *will* be repositioned during surgery.
- **Skin loss** - due to impaired circulation and aggrivated by smoking, may require secondary surgery to improve scar appearance.

These are only some of the risks and complications that should be considered when making the decision to undergo tummy tuck surgery. You should discuss this subject in detail with your surgeon and his staff, and be fully aware of the risks and possible complications prior to signing your consent form.

PREOPERATIVE INSTRUCTIONS

At the time that you schedule your procedure, either the doctor or someone on his staff will review with you some instructions that you should follow in the days or weeks immediately prior to your surgery, as well as for the day that your procedure is to be done. Some of the more common items that most surgeons will include are:

- Do not take any medication containing aspirin for up to two weeks prior to surgery (can cause excessive bleeding). In addition, your surgeon may recommend that you discontinue use of some hormone medications, birth control pills and certain vitamin supplements - *check with your doctor*!
- The surgeon may advise that the patient take additional Vitamin C for a few days prior to surgery, and some surgeons may prescribe an antibiotic to be taken for a specified number of days before surgery.
- Stop cigarette smoking - it affects healing and may contribute to scarring, etc. No alcoholic beverages up to forty-eight hours prior to surgery.
- Nothing to eat or drink after midnight the night before surgery.
- Arrange for someone to drive you to and from the hospital, as well as a responsible adult to be with you for at least the first few days following your release from the hospital.

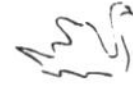

Finally, have a supply of "quiet" activities on hand to keep you busy for the first week of your recovery. Reading, television, needle work, etc. will help you pass the time. Try to avoid excitement and visitors for the first few days. Be certain that you understand all of the instructions given to you; call your surgeon's office if you are confused at all.

THE TUMMY TUCK PROCEDURE

Since the vast majority of abdominoplasty procedures are performed on an inpatient basis, you may be asked to check in to the hospital the night before your surgery is scheduled. At the latest, you will probably have to report in at least a couple of hours prior to your operation. Once there, you may have some minor preliminary tests done (such as blood typing, etc.) followed by a meeting with the anesthesiologist. The anesthesiologist will ask you some questions to assure that you are a good candidate for general anesthesia - ***be certain to answer these questions completely and honestly.***

Just prior to surgery you'll most likely have an IV placed in your arm or wrist which will be used to facilitate the administration of fluids and medication during surgery, and you may be given a mild sedative to help you to relax. The surgeon will also draw his surgical "roadmap" on your tummy, the lines and arrows and circles which will help guide his incisions and navel placement during the operation.

After all the preparations have been made, you'll lie down on the operating table, where cardiac monitors will probably be taped to your chest and upper back. Just before the surgeon is ready to begin a heavier sedation will probably be administered by way of your IV tube (or injection). This sedation will relax you to the point that you begin to "nap", and the anesthesiologist will begin the general anesthesia.

Once you are well "under" the anesthesia and the abdominal area has been thoroughly cleansed with a strong antibacterial soap, the surgeon will begin making his incisions. If liposuction will be used during your procedure, the small incisions made to insert the canula (suction tube) will probably be made first, through which the surgeon will remove the appropriate amount of fatty tissue. Be certain to read the chapter on liposuction so that you better understand this process, as well as the accompanying benefits and possible complications.

The incisions most commonly made for the tummy tuck run virtually the width of the lower abdomen, in the natural creases where the legs meet the torso, and up across the area directly above the pubic area. The surgeon will also cut around the navel, leaving the underlying supporting tissues attached.

When the large incision is made the skin and fat will be separated from the underlying layer of muscle, exposing the covering of the abdominal muscles. Some of the muscles that help hold the abdomen firm, the *rectus abdominus*, lie within the area that will be exposed. These muscles may become separated during pregnancy, and the surgeon may determine that it is necessary to reinforce the abdomen by surgically rejoining these muscles.

Once the work has been done on the muscles, the detached flap of skin and fat will be pulled downward, toward the pubic area. The redundant skin and fat will then be cut away and the navel "threaded" through the incision made at its new location. Of course, any pre-existing scars or stretch marks that lie within the area of skin to be removed will be gone after surgery, along with the excess skin and fat.

The incisions will most likely be sutured closed with the patient in a slightly bent position. This removes any stress or tension on the suture site, and will help in the healing process. The navel will be stitched in its new position as well, with the sutures lying within the "belly button".

Be aware that severely obese patients or patients with a great deal of excess skin may require additional incisions, or incisions made at different locations than the procedure described above. In some cases, an incision may be made all the way around the waistline, and/or a "T" shaped incision may be necessary, with the vertical part of the "T" running the length of the tummy. Naturally, the resulting scars from these incisions will be much more extensive. The patient must consider this scarring in the decision-making process, and then proceed with the surgery fully aware of the probable results.

Throughout the operation the surgeon will be dealing with bleeding. He will use an electrical device called a *cauterizer* to seal the blood vessels. Normally, the operation will take from three to four hours, but if excessive bleeding occurs the surgery can take longer.

Once all of the incisions are closed, the surgeon or nurse will apply gauze bandages to the affected area, with surgical tape covering the gauze. In addition, most surgeons will put you in either elastic bandages or some other firm supporting undergarment to help support the area during recovery.

You will then be wheeled out to a recovery area, where the anesthesiologist and hospital staff will monitor your immediate postoperative recovery. When you are able, you will be moved to your hospital room for further rest and recovery, probably after an hour or two. Plan on a total hospital stay of two to four days for the tummy tuck surgery and recovery.

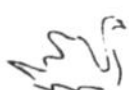

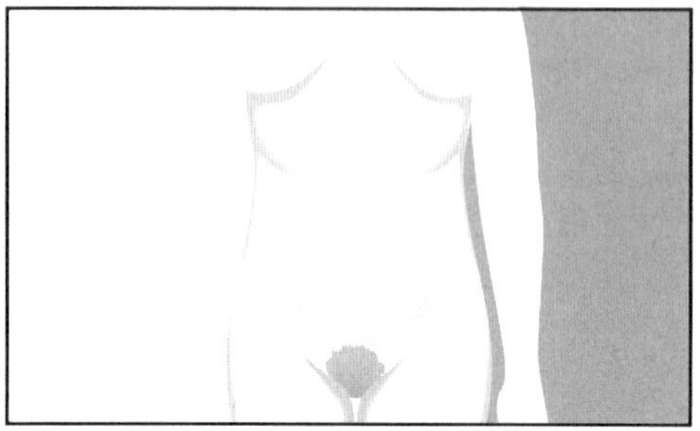

Preoperative tummy tuck patient with excess skin and fat in the abdominal area.

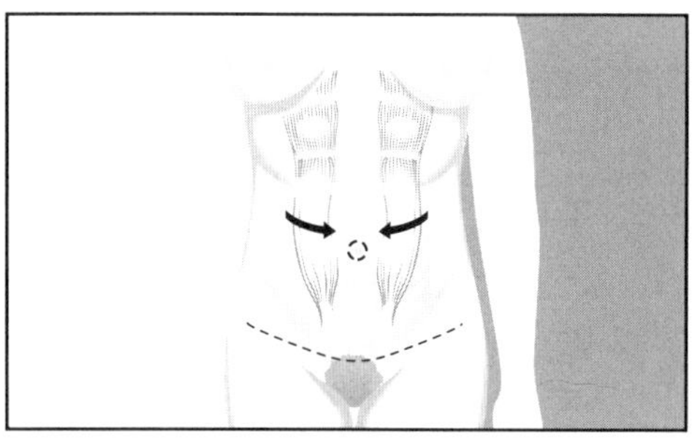

Incisions will commonly extend horizontally across the lower abdomen above the pubic area. A circular incision is made around the navel. The surgeon may suture the abdominal muscle together to tighten the abdomen.

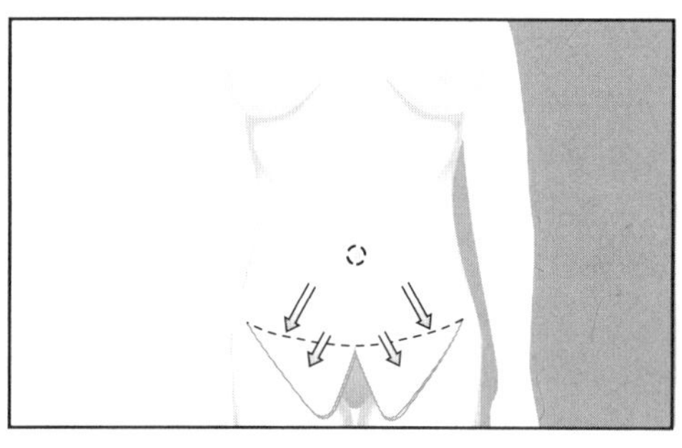

Skin and fat tissue is pulled downward toward the pubic area. The redundant skin and fat is removed.

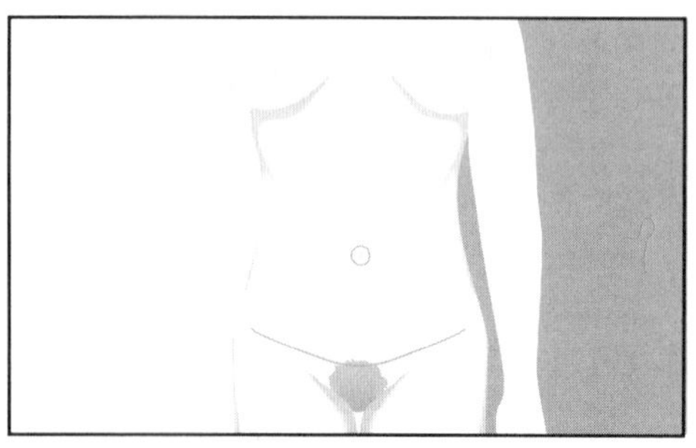

Postoperative tummy tuck patient with a firmer, flatter abdomen. Scars extend horizontally across the lower abdomen above the pubic area.

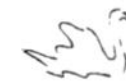

THE RECOVERY PERIOD

During the two or three days that you will be recovering in the hospital, you should expect to experience some discomfort and pain. For the first day or two, nurses will probably give you pain medication by injection. For the remainder of your recovery at home you'll most likely receive a prescription pain reliever that can be taken as needed, and as directed. You may have a catheter in place that was positioned before surgery; some surgeons will leave it in for a day or so, since the patient may have trouble getting up and down to go to the bathroom. The small drains placed in your abdomen during surgery to help express any blood and fluids will be removed within two to three days after the operation. Some surgeons will restrict bathing while stitches are in, others will allow you to shower or bathe and reapply clean gauze bandages yourself.

Most doctors will want you up and moving around as soon as possible, since extensive bed rest can increase your chances of developing phlebitis (inflammation of the veins, especially in the leg). You will probably walk in a stooped position for a few days - the tension on your lower abdomen by standing fully upright may be uncomfortable and stress the incisions. You will probably be advised to sleep on your side (in the fetal position) or on your back with pillows placed beneath your knees to reduce the tension on the affected area. Sleeping on your tummy will be out of the question for a month or so. In addition, most people feel extremely fatigued and tire easily for up to a couple of weeks after surgery - due, in part, to the use of general anesthesia. It will be at least two weeks before you will be up to returning to work, longer if you had more extensive surgery or if you have an active type job. Sex can be resumed after about three weeks, while sports and other heavy activity will have to wait six weeks or more.

The supporting undergarments (like a surgical or panty girdle) will be worn for four to six weeks. The gauze and tape beneath the girdle will remain in place for a couple of weeks, usually until all of the stitches are out. If deep sutures were used to pull together your abdominal muscles, they will be permanent. Most of the other stitches are removed within two weeks, depending on the type of sutures that were used. Expect some swelling and bruising for at least a couple of weeks. You can anticipate a slight degree of swelling to persist for up to six months or more.

RESULTS

As we have said previously in the chapter, the results of the tummy tuck are permanent, in that the fat and skin removed during the procedure do not reappear. The abdomen will appear flatter and more taut after the tummy tuck. Excess skin and fat, as well as muscle weakening can recur, however, if a pregnancy or substantial weight gain/loss transpires after surgery. Since some postoperative

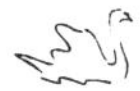

swelling can persist for a period of months, don't be too hasty in judging the effectiveness of your tummy tuck. You should plan on waiting six months or so before seeing the full result of your procedure.

The scars resulting from your surgery are permanent, and some patients will experience wide, bright pink or raised scarring. Some treatment for unsightly scarring is available, such as steroid treatment, but they may not always be effective. You must decide if the trade-off of scarring versus a sagging abdomen is worth it to you.

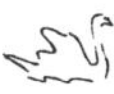

CHAPTER TEN

LIPOSUCTION

"Oh who can tell the range of joy

Or set the bounds of beauty?"

Sara Teasdale
"A Winter Bluejay", *River to the Sea* (1915)

Rebecca is a highly energetic mother of two who manages to run her own business out of her home, play tennis on a ladie's league twice a week and keep up with a busy, active family. At five-foot-six, she appears fashionably slim in an athletic sort-of way, dressed in nice jeans and a lovely sweater. After my comment that she doesn't look like anyone who ever had needed the procedure known as ***"fat suctioning"****, she laughs out loud.*

Reaching into her sizeable purse, she pulls out a small pile of photographs and pushes them across the table in my direction. "Take a look for yourself," she says, with a knowing grin.

As I look through the photos, I readily recognize her face and the honey-blonde hair right away. But the body in those pictures was not the same as the one sitting across from me now. The person in the photographs had large round hips and appeared much heavier. Acknowledging the changes, I asked her how much weight she had lost in addition to having liposuction. "You're going to have trouble believing this," she said. "But my weight hasn't changed by more than three or four pounds since I've had my children."

She was right. It was hard to believe that she hadn't lost a good ten or twelve pounds since those pictures were taken. Then she pulled out her "before and after" pictures, taken by the cosmetic surgeon who had performed her liposuction. Looking at those photographs, it was immediately obvious as to what was to blame for her previously heavy appearance. She had large "bags" of excess fat on her hips and upper thighs (what is commonly referred to as saddlebags). Obviously, Rebecca was very pleased with the results of her liposuction.

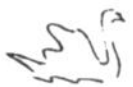

Liposuction has taken the cosmetic surgery world by storm. It seems that almost everyone has some problem area or another that they want to disappear. According to data gathered by the American Society of Plastic and Reconstructive Surgeons from its members, over a hundred thousand liposuction procedures were performed by members of that group in 1990 alone. In just a relatively few short years, it has become the most popular cosmetic procedure.

While the majority of liposuction patients are women, 10 percent of the people who underwent liposuction in 1990 were men. Most of these liposuction patients are fairly young: **88 percent** were under age 50. This can be partly attributed to one of the physical characteristics that make up a good liposuction candidate - the skin must have good elasticity in order to adjust favorably to the new contour of the underlying tissues (more on that later).

Liposuction (or ***suction-assisted lipectomy or lipolysis***) is used on various parts of the body: on the face and neck during a facelift, on the abdomen during a tummy tuck, on the arms, knees and buttocks. The most popular spot for fat suctioning, though, is the hips and thighs with 42 percent of the 1990 liposuction procedures directed at these problem areas.

As wonderful as it sounds, make no mistake about liposuction - it is surgery. And it has limitations, risks and possible complications. Contrary to what you may have heard, liposuction *will not* get rid of cellulite, nor is it a replacement for a healthy diet and regular exercise program or a solution to obesity. **Liposuction is best used to remove localized areas of excess fat that are resistant to diet and exercise**.

WHO IS A CANDIDATE FOR LIPOSUCTION?

Ideally, liposuction patients are in good general health, have maintained a stable weight that is suitable for their body build, have no history of phlebitis (inflammation of the veins), and have a level of skin elasticity that will allow the skin to adapt well to the new surgically-altered contour. Since no skin is removed during the liposuction procedure, elasticity of the skin is of primary concern, after the criteria regarding the health, expectations and motivation of the patient. Obviously, patients who expect liposuction alone to change their lives or save their marriage will be sadly disappointed. This procedure, as with all cosmetic surgery, should be undertaken with *improvement* rather than perfection as the goal. If the results of the surgery help you to feel better about yourself, your life may, indeed, improve. But it will be because of a boost to your self-esteem and self-image, not because of the results of the procedure itself.

Skin elasticity will be less of a factor if liposuction is being done as part of a procedure in which skin is being removed, as in a facelift or tummy tuck. Many

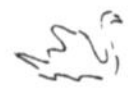

cosmetic surgeons are incorporating liposuction into these types of procedures on a routine basis, and with very favorable results.

Your plastic surgeon will, of course, do a full evaluation of your condition at the time of consultation. Some of the things that he or she will be looking at are:

- Your overall health
- Skin Elasticity
- Muscle tone
- Body Build
- Skin type and coloring
- Amount of localized fat to be removed
- Medical history
- Weight

Again, it is important that the patient realize that liposuction is *not* intended to cure obesity or replace a healthy regimen of diet and exercise. The ideal patient will be at a stable, healthy weight for his or her height and build.

ANESTHESIA

A high percentage of plastic surgeons will recommend that the liposuction procedure be done at an outpatient surgical center or in his own surgical facility. Anesthesia will depending on the size of the area to be treated: for treating small, localized areas the surgeon may recommend sedation and local anesthetics administered by a nurse or the doctor himself. With heavy sedation you will not be unconscious during surgery but you will most likely be sedated to a degree that you "nap" throughout the procedure. ***A word to the wise about anesthesia: even if your surgeon feels that a physician anesthesiologist is not necessary for your surgery, you have a right to discuss your options. It will incur additional expense, but the added security of having a trained doctor just monitoring your overall condition during the procedure can be well worth the money. Remember, the surgeon will be busy performing the operation. A substantial quantity of body fluids can be lost during liposuction, and one of the responsibilities of the anesthesiologist is to monitor the replacement of those fluids and to assure your physical well-being.***

To remove the possibility of physical discomfort in the areas to be treated, a local anesthetic will be administered after the sedation has had time to make you relaxed. The prick of the needle and subsequent burning or stinging sensation as the local anesthetic is injected may be slightly uncomfortable, but will soon be replaced by numbness in the area.

In procedures involving a larger area to be treated, the doctor may consider it necessary to use general anesthesia. If this is true in your case, make certain that the person administering the general anesthesia is either a physician anesthesiologist or a certified nurse anesthetist. With this type of anesthesia, you

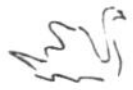

will be placed in an unconscious state for the duration of the surgery. Be certain to read Chapter Two concerning the risks and complications associated with anesthesia.

COST

The expense associated with your liposuction procedure can vary to a substantial degree, depending on what type of surgical facility your plastic surgeon chooses to utilize, how long of a hospital stay is necessary for your operation, and the normal fees charged by surgeons in your geographical area. Most liposuction procedures are being done on an outpatient basis; only 13 percent of the liposuction surgeries performed by members of the ASPRS in 1990 were done on an inpatient basis.

The anesthesia of choice for your operation will be a factor in your final cost, as well. General anesthesia is almost always administered by a physician anesthesiologist whose fees are separate and above those charged by the surgeon, while local anesthesia with sedation is frequently administered by a nurse or the surgeon himself.

The **average** surgeon's fees for single-site (both of your hips or both legs would be considered a single-site, while a surgery in which tummy and hips were done probably would not) liposuction procedures done in 1990 by members of the American Society of Plastic and Reconstructive Surgeons were:

LOW	AVERAGE	HIGH
$500	**$1480**	**$5000**

Again, you should be aware that surgeon's fees will differ throughout geographic regions of the country. In general, prices are somewhat higher on the east and west coasts, with the least expensive fees available in the interior regions of the United States. These are generalities and should not be used to measure the fees charged by your surgeon. Make certain that you discuss *all* of the costs involved for your procedure prior to surgery day, including anesthesiologist fees, post-operative care, hospital costs, etc.

As with most cosmetic procedures, the cost of liposuction is not usually covered by health insurance if undergone for strictly aesthetic reasons. Most surgeons will want payment of their fees prior to surgery. Find out in advance what arrangements need to be made with the hospital and anesthesiologist. Some hospitals have a very lenient repayment schedule, others do not, requiring

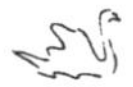

immediate payment. Discuss this in detail with your surgeon's staff, the anesthesiologist's office and the hospital.

RISKS AND COMPLICATIONS

Aside from the risks associated with the anesthesia (review Chapter Two), there are several risks, possible complications and draw-backs that should be considered when making the decision to undergo liposuction surgery:

- **Bleeding** - any surgery that involves areas containing blood vessels includes the risk of excessive bleeding.
- **Hematoma** - is, basically, bleeding beneath the skin. If the bleeding does not subside fairly quickly, the surgeon may have to reoperate remove the blood. Small hematomas can sometimes be taken care of without second surgery by expressing the blood with a syringe.
- **Scarring** - from liposuction is usually a fairly minor concern, since the incisions necessary to insert the suction tube (*cannula*) are relatively small.
- **Numbness** - can be experienced in the treated areas. Feeling generally returns within a few weeks. In rare cases, numbness can take months or even years to subside, or can be permanent.
- **Infection** - the risk of infection always exists in surgery. The surgeon will prescribe antibiotics in an effort to prevent infection, but it does occur in rare cases. Infection can cause many complications in healing, and can be an extremely serious, life-threatening problem.
- **Abnormal pigmentation** - is experienced by some patients following the liposuction procedure. This is usually seen as localized "blotchy" areas of darker pigmentation in the treated areas.
- **Pain** - is to be expected in the first two or three days after surgery. The doctor will most likely give you a prescription for pain medication for your initial recovery period at home, up to a few days or so. Expect to experience aching and soreness in the treated areas for up to a few weeks.
- **Seroma** - is a collection of fluids in the hollowed-out areas where the fat was suctioned. Most occurrences of a seroma can be treated by the doctor expressing the fluid with a syringe. Rarely, a second operation will be necessary to remove the fluids.
- **Fat or blood clots** - It is possible that fat dislodged during the procedure could enter the bloodstream and cause difficulty to vital organs. Phlebitis, or blood clot in the legs, has been seen following surgical procedures. Again, should the clot become dislodged, it could cause difficulty in the normal function of vital organs, even death in rare cases.

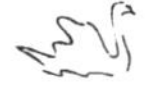

- **Waviness, Ridges, Bumps and Uneven healing** - are commonly seen in liposuction results. If too much or too little fat is suctioned, the treated area can have a rippled appearance, or a ridge can be seen where the suctioned area meets the untreated area. Waviness can be caused by adhesions that form in the healing process, and by scarring within the tissue.
- **Hypovolemia** - is rare, and is caused by the depletion of fluids in the body, can result in the patient going into shock. This is one of the reasons that it is a good idea to have an anesthesiologist on hand for the procedure, since he will be monitoring (along with the surgeon) the proper replacement of the fluids that are lost during the liposuction procedure.
- **Muscle and organ damage** - while rare, the possibility does exist for the suction tube to in advertently damage the muscles or organs adjoining the fatty areas being treated.

These are only some of the risks and complications that should be considered when making the decision to undergo liposuction. You should discuss this subject in detail with your surgeon and his staff, and be fully aware of the risks and possible complications prior to signing your consent form.

PREOPERATIVE INSTRUCTIONS

At the time that you schedule your procedure, either the doctor or someone on his staff will review with you some instructions that you should follow in the days or weeks immediately prior to your surgery, as well as for the day that your procedure is to be done. Some of the more common items that most surgeons will include are:

- Do not take any medication containing aspirin for up to two weeks prior to surgery (can cause excessive bleeding). In addition, your surgeon may recommend that you discontinue use of some hormone medications, birth control pills and certain vitamin supplements - ***check with your doctor!***
- The surgeon may advise that the patient take additional Vitamin C for a few days prior to surgery, and some surgeons may prescribe an antibiotic to be taken for a specified number of days before surgery.
- Stop cigarette smoking - it affects healing and may contribute to scarring, etc.
- No alcoholic beverages up to forty-eight hours prior to surgery.
- Nothing to eat or drink after midnight the night before surgery.
- Arrange for someone to drive you to and from the hospital or surgical center, as well as a responsible adult to be with you for the twenty-four hours following your release from the doctor's care.

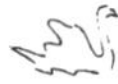

Finally, have a supply of "quiet" activities on hand to keep you busy for the first week of your recovery. Reading, television, needle work, etc. will help you pass the time. Try to avoid excitement and visitors for the first few days. Be certain that you understand all of the instructions given to you; call your surgeon's office if you are at all confused.

THE LIPOSUCTION PROCEDURE

If your liposuction procedure is to be performed on an inpatient basis, you may be asked to check in to the hospital the night before your surgery. At the latest, you will probably have to report in at least a couple of hours prior to your operation. Once at the hospital, you may have some minor preliminary tests done (such as blood work, etc.) followed by a meeting with the anesthesiologist. The anesthesiologist will ask you some questions to assure that you are a good candidate for general anesthesia - ***be certain to answer these questions completely and honestly.***

For procedures done on an outpatient basis, you'll probably be asked to arrive an hour or so before surgery. As with the surgery done in the hospital, you'll probably meet with the anesthesiologist and have some minor lab work done.

Just prior to surgery you'll most likely have an IV placed in your arm or wrist which will be used to facilitate the administration of fluids and medication during surgery, and you may be given a mild sedative to help you to relax. The surgeon will also draw his surgical "roadmap" on the area to be treated during surgery, the lines and arrows and circles which will help guide his incisions and suctioning during the operation.

After all the preparations have been made you'll lie down on the operating table, where cardiac monitors will probably be taped to your chest and upper back. Just before the surgeon is ready to begin a heavier sedation will probably be administered by way of your IV tube (or injection). This sedation will relax you to the point that you begin to "nap". If you are to have general anesthesia, the anesthesiologist will begin it now.

Once you are well "under" the anesthesia and the areas to be treated have been thoroughly cleansed with a strong antibacterial soap, the surgeon will begin making his first incision. The incisions necessary for liposuction are relatively small, usually no longer than an inch or so, and serve as an entry point into the body through which the surgeon will insert the cannula (suction tube).

After inserting the suction tube into the area to be treated, the surgeon will vigorously move the tube back and forth, suctioning fat as he goes. Small tunnels are formed under the skin from the removal of the fat. It is because of these tunnels that the proper replacement of body fluids is so important in the liposuction

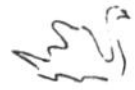

procedure, since the body will rush fluids to the treated areas in an attempt to fill the empty tunnels. The amount of suctioning will, of course, depend on the amount of fat to be removed. The maximum **total amount** that can be safely removed in one session will differ from patient to patient. Excessive removal will put the patient at risk for hypovolemia, or the dangerous depletion of body fluids. These hollowed-out areas are also why some patients can experience a rippling effect in the suctioned area, as well as bumps and ridges in the tissue beneath the skin.

After all the areas to be treated have been suctioned, the surgeon will suture the small incisions made for inserting the cannula. You'll be fitted into a support garment at this point, the type depending on what part of your body was treated. For the area between the waist and the knees, a long panty or surgical girdle will be necessary. For other areas an elastic support bandage of some sort may be adequate. Most liposuction procedures take from an hour or so up to three hours, depending on how much work is to be done.

After the procedure is complete, you'll be moved into a postoperative recovery area, where the staff and anesthesiologist will monitor your immediate recovery. Depending on the amount of fat removed in the session, you may be allowed to go home after an hour or so. If a large volume of fat was suctioned you may be required to spend the night under medical supervision before being released.

THE RECOVERY PERIOD

Expect to be sore in the treated area for a couple of weeks, with the more severe discomfort taking place in the first few days after surgery. Most surgeons will prescribe a mild pain medication to be taken as needed for a week or so. The average patient will feel up to returning to a non-active type job by around the fifth day after surgery, but the doctor will probably want you to remain as immobile as possible for the first one to four days after the procedure. More vigorous activity should be postponed for up to three weeks. Ask your surgeon about any specific activities that you are concerned about.

Extensive swelling and bruising will be present for a couple of weeks - most of it diminishing by week three or four after surgery. Some small degree of swelling can persist for a matter of months, so give your results time to become fully apparent.

The stitches that were required to close the small incisions made during your surgery will be removed within a week or so. Very small scars may remain, but should be inconspicuous.

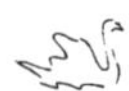

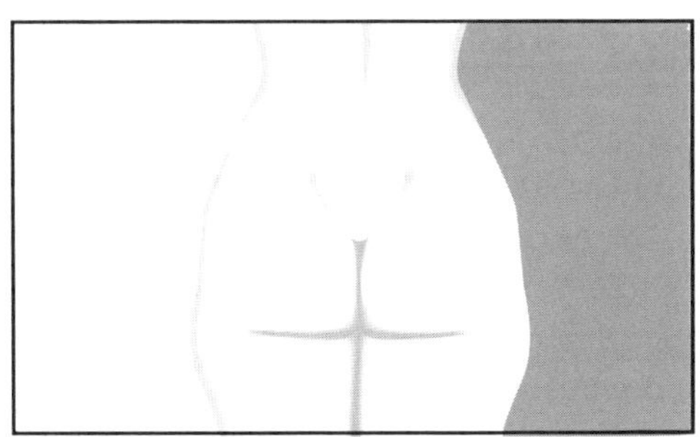

Preoperative liposuction patient with prominent localized fat on thighs.

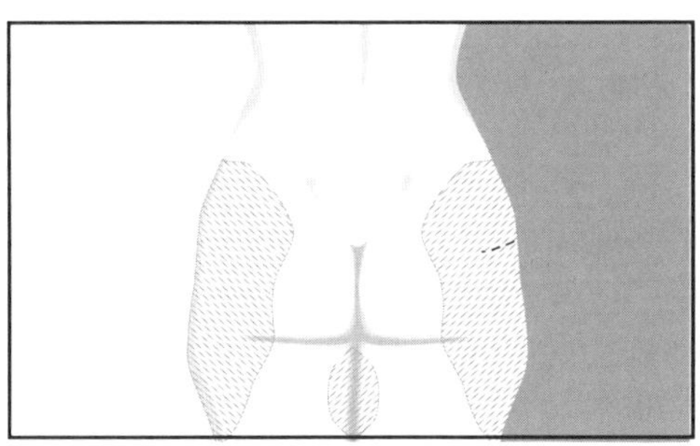

A small incision is made to insert the suction instrument for removal of the fat. The shading represents areas commonly treated with liposuction.

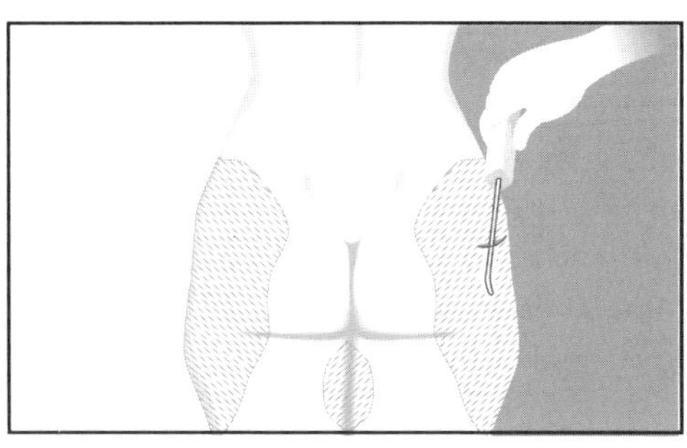

The suction instrument is inserted through the skin and moved back and forth within the area to be treated.

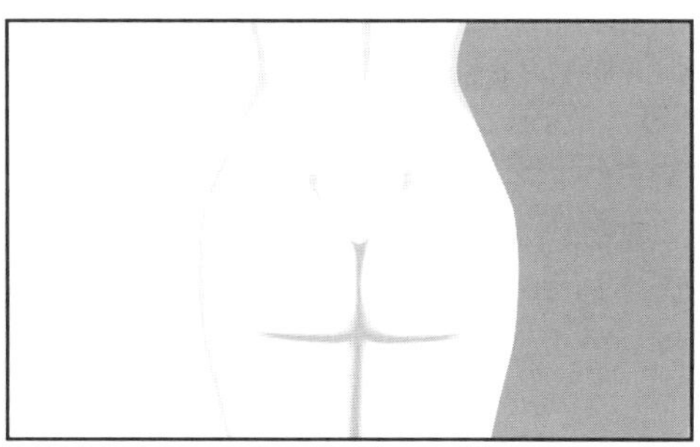

Postoperative liposuction patient with prominent localized fatty areas removed, resulting in a smoother body contour.

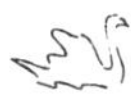

Before you leave the operating room, you'll be placed in a support garment. The length of time that you'll be required to keep these elastic bandages on will depend on the site and extent of the suctioning. Most facial liposuction patients can stop wearing the elastic support within a week after surgery, while those who had fat suctioned in the abdomen, hips, thighs or buttocks will probably have to remain in the support garment (like a girdle) for up to three weeks or so. This support or *compression* garment is very important to the healing process, since it will help the skin to conform to the new contours created by the suction procedure. For the first few days after surgery the garment will remain in place at all times (specially made to allow you to go to the bathroom). This is not only to help the redraping of the skin, but also to help alleviate the build-up of fluids (blood or serum) in the treated tissues. After the first postoperative visit to the doctor, you'll probably be allowed to take it off for cleaning and to take your shower or bath. At your last postoperative checkup, the surgeon will advise you as to how long the garment should continue to be worn. Don't be tempted to skimp on wearing your support garment - its purpose is to help maximize your results and assure proper healing!

Most surgeons will also recommend a regimen of massage for the treated areas, to begin within a few days after surgery. Many doctors fell that water-jet or hot tub type massage is also recommended.

RESULTS

Most patients who go into liposuction with realistic expectations are pleased with their results, bearing in mind that the goal in liposuction is to ***bring areas of localized excess fat into proportion with the rest of the body***. Patients who have cellulite before liposuction will have it afterward, and it may sometimes be even more noticeable after the surgery. Remember that the procedure itself can occasionally cause dimpling and rippling of the skin, caused by the tunneling made by the fat suctioning, as well as contour irregularities.

The results of liposuction can be considered permanent, since the fat cells removed during surgery are gone forever. There is some disagreement as to whether the suctioned areas are less susceptible to new fat. Most doctors feel that the treated areas will remain in proportion to the rest of the body. That is, if you put on weight after surgery, you'll gain fat proportionately all over, rather than being localized in the problem area (as may have been the case prior to treatment).

As with any procedure, new liposuction techniques are constantly being developed and refined. Dr. J. Barry Boyd, a Winter Park (Florida) plastic surgeon, has made several recent changes in his suction lipectomy (liposuction) techniques

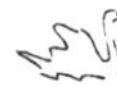

which he feels improve both results and recovery. Some of the changes that he mentions are improved patient pre-operative preparation, new positioning techniques and cooling the surgical area before and after suction. As liposuction goes through its refining stages patients should begin to see better results and improved methods of dealing with unwanted side-effects, such as dimpling and rippling.

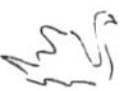

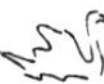

CHAPTER ELEVEN

CHEMICAL PEELS

"Living well and beautifully and justly are all one thing."

Socrates
In Plato's Crito (*4th c.* B.C.)
tr. Lane Cooper

Americans have a fixation with youth. We all want to look young, feel young and think young. Unfortunately, Father Time has a different agenda. As we age, our skin begins to give evidence to those wonderful summers at the beach, the weekends spent playing tennis or golf in the bright sunshine, and all of the accumulated hours that we've spent squinting into the harsh sunlight.

How Our Skin Ages

In fact, the damage caused by exposure to sunlight is the primary factor in bringing about the first visible signs of aging skin. As we get older (though sometimes as soon as our late twenties or early thirties) the substance which binds the outer layers of our skin begins to adhere these layers too tightly together. The outermost surface of the skin, or ***stratum corneum***, begins to thicken and shrink. As this occurs the skin can take on a dry, rough, scaly appearance with an uneven or "sallow" skin tone. Pores become more prominent, areas of uneven pigmentation (usually referred to as "age spots") can crop up, as well as incidents of adult acne. At the onset of these symptoms most people begin to notice that their skin feels dry and tight, and begin using moisturizers and skin conditioners in earnest. The primary function of these skin care products is to reduce the *symptoms* of the

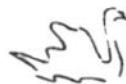

condition, relieving the tightness and dry feeling. Unfortunately, the damage has already been done and all of the moisturizer in the world will not undo the effects of prior sun damage.

The second set of visible signs of sun-induced aging are fine lines and wrinkles, caused by a collapse in the *dermis* (underlying layers of skin). This collapse occurs when the levels of collagen and elastin in the skin tissues are depleted and the skin surface looses its underlying support system.

There are other forces at work on your skin, and therefore your appearance. Namely, *gravity*. Gravity, as you well know, maintains a constant downward pull on every object on earth. This is very good news if you aren't in the mood to go drifting off into space, but bad news for our anatomy. This same downward pull also acts on our skin and other tissues, causing sags, bags and pouches to appear as our skin ages and we lose some of the skin elasticity that we enjoyed in our youth. ***Chemical peels are* not *effective treatment for sagging skin.*** These pouches and bags of loose skin are best treated with a surgical procedure, such as a facelift or blepharoplasty (eyelid surgery).

What does all of this mean to you? It means that usually by the time you reach your forties, you have begun to notice dry scaly skin, an uneven or "sallow" complexion, and the onset of fine lines and wrinkles (especially in the area of the eyes and mouth). What can you do about it? Well, some people decide to pay a visit to their cosmetic surgeon for answers. One of the possible treatments that your surgeon may suggest is the ***chemical peel.***

According to data gathered by the ASPRS from its members, the number of patients undergoing the chemical peel procedure increased 46 percent between 1988 and 1990. Most surgeons attribute the dramatic increase to a greater awareness and acceptance of cosmetic surgery on the part of the public, and to the introduction of new substances and techniques used in the chemical peel process. Recent developments and new technology have set the aesthetic surgery world abuzz, with new and exciting changes in the substances and methodology being used in the fight against aging, sun-damaged skin. With these changes, the types of patients and skin conditions that can be treated with a chemical peel have expanded dramatically. The cosmetic surgeon has gained a great deal of flexibility and control in the peel process. Patients with darker skin were not previously good candidates for a chemical peel in the past, since the substance used also lightened or bleached the skin, causing a marked difference in skin color between the treated areas and those which had not been affected by the peel. The substance most commonly used in the past for a chemical peel was an extremely potent, potentially toxic chemical called ***phenol***. While there are still some conditions that are treated more successfully with phenol, this substance has some serious complications, risks and drawbacks, which will be discussed later in this chapter.

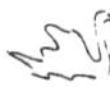

There are a number of substances that are being used in new ways and in new concentrations that are so effective in the chemical peel process that they are quickly becoming the chemicals of choice for many cosmetic surgeons. By far, the chemical currently creating the biggest stir among this group of medical professionals is ***trichloroacetic-acid***, or TCA. TCA has proven effective for use on patients with dark skin, and it is thought not to be absorbed through the skin into the system, reducing the chances of potential toxicity. In addition, it can be used on areas of the body other than the face with pleasing results. Many medical professionals are referring to the TCA peel as a "***rejuvenation peel***".

How Chemical Peels Work

For years, plastic surgeons have used chemical agents in an attempt to beautify the appearance. Applied to the skin in very controlled concentrations and for very specific periods of time, these chemicals (acids, actually) react with the skin surface and create a mild "burn". After a short period of time (depending on the type of acid used), the skin treated with the chemical will *slough*, or peel off, revealing the healthier, smoother and younger-looking skin beneath.

Do not make the mistake of taking a chemical peel lightly, however. This is not as simple as applying a mud mask to your face and washing it off a few minutes later. These are acids that literally remove the top layer of your skin. Some of the acids are potentially toxic, and can cause serious health problems if not administered properly by an experienced medical professional. Beware of advertisements promoting "skin rejuvenation" and "non-surgical facelifts" to be performed by **non-medical** professionals. Be absolutely certain that you select treatment that is administered by a licensed, board-certified medical professional, such as a plastic surgeon.

With the new chemical solutions and techniques gaining popularity in the peel process, plastic surgeons have a greater variety of treatment available to their patients. A patient in her mid thirties, for example, may be just beginning to see the signs of sun damage to her skin, manifested by a rough, scaly appearance and a poor complexion tone. Obviously, this person is not quite ready for a full **deep** chemical peel. In a case such as this the cosmetic surgeon may recommend a **light or medium** TCA peel, which is a much more superficial treatment than the deeper TCA or phenol peel. It should, however, be adequate to alleviate the patient's problems with skin tone, fine lines, uneven pigmentation (age spots) and the rough, scaly appearance of the outer skin layer.

Since a light chemical peel does not remove deep tissues (it serves primarily to slough the stratum corneum) and has a much shorter recovery period (usually no more than a week to ten days), it can be repeated every couple of weeks or so,

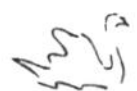

if necessary. In treating a patient with repetitive light peels, the plastic surgeon can control the peel process much more effectively than when using a single deep peel. He can treat specific problem areas repeatedly in a short period of time, and in a localized fashion. If that fairly young patient is happy with the results of the first light peel but still has areas of uneven pigmentation, for example, the surgeon can apply the chemical solution only to those areas needing further treatment. Be aware, however, that extremely light concentrations of TCA may produce results that last only a few months, and repeated treatments within a short period of time may cause temporary irritation.

Patients exhibiting more pronounced signs of aging skin, such as deeper wrinkles and "lipstick" lines around the mouth, may require a deeper peel in order to enjoy the results that they are looking for. These deeper peels are usually done utilizing either a stronger concentration of TCA, or with phenol. A deeper peel will improve skin tone, uneven pigmentation, remove fine lines, smooth the skin surface, vastly improve complexion tone and soften deep wrinkles.

Deeper peels generally have more swelling and redness of the skin postoperatively, and have a slightly longer recovery period. Deep TCA peels generally take up to ten days or two weeks for recovery, while recovery from a phenol peel may take up to a month or more. As a rule, the deeper the peel, the more potential that exists for negative side effects and complications.

Obviously, the condition of your skin will determine the depth and type of chemical peel that your plastic surgeon will recommend. In the next few pages, we'll give you a general idea of the methodology, recovery, results and risks or complications associated with the types of chemical peels most commonly used by cosmetic surgeons.

PREPARING THE SKIN FOR A CHEMICAL PEEL

One of the advances that plastic surgeons have made in recent years is the realization that the preparation of the skin prior to the peel is of utmost importance in improving the results of the treatment. It is fairly common practice now for the surgeon to start a patient (**up to six weeks prior to the peel)** on a substance which will improve the penetration of the chemical into the skin. Improved penetration of a milder chemical solution can give the patient equal or better results than a peel done with a stronger concentration, with fewer potential complications. Some of the substances that your doctor may use in his preparation process are synthetic vitamin A derivatives or **alpha-hydroxy acids**.

Vitamin A derivatives, of course, has received much publicity of late as a treatment for the signs of aging in sun-damaged skin. These treatments act on the outer layer of skin, promoting the sloughing off of the thickened skin. Removal of

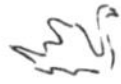

this thickened barrier prior to the application of the chemical peel solution allows the acid to penetrate more quickly and more evenly. Some surgeons may recommend that **hydroquinone** (a bleaching substance) be combined in the preparation treatment; it serves to help avoid areas of uneven pigmentation after the peel, especially in patients with darker complexions.

Products containing **glycolic acid** are also being used as a pre-peel skin preparation. Glycolic acid is an *alpha-hydroxy acid* found in sugar cane, and is gaining rapid acceptance among cosmetic surgeons and dermatologists as an alternative (or supplement) for vitamin A derivatives. Like its vitamin A counterpart, glycolic acid weakens the outer skin layer and promotes the shedding of the dead skin cells. The stratum corneum (outer-most layer of skin) sloughs off, and the smoother, healthier underlying skin is revealed. Some of the reasons cited for the increasing popularity of glycolic acid products are as follows: increased penetration and greater effectiveness due to a smaller molecular structure, less irritation and sun-sensitivity, and indications that glycolic acid may help regenerate collagen and elastin in the dermis (depletion of collagen and elastin contributes to the onset of deeper wrinkles caused by sun damage). Some plastic surgeons will use an alpha-hydroxy acid as an additive to the chemical peel solution, or as an application immediately prior to the peel solution, as well.

Most surgeons will lower the concentration of the chemical peel solution when a patient has been using one of these preparation substances. The chemical peel and these products share a unique relationship - they each enhance the effectiveness of the other. Many surgeons and patients feel that, following a chemical peel, the results obtained by using vitamin A derivatives or alpha-hydroxy acid products are much improved. We will discuss the post-peel skin care regimen later in this chapter.

THE LIGHT TO MEDIUM CHEMICAL PEEL

The best candidates for light to medium peels are those patients who are noticing the onset of symptoms of sun-damaged aging skin. These symptoms would include a rough, scaly appearance to the skin, fine lines and wrinkles around the eyes, chin and lips, and a sallow, ruddy, dull cast to the complexion. Also, patients with precancerous lesions (localized areas of roughly textured abnormal pigmentation) are effectively treated with a light to medium peel. The most common chemical of choice currently used by plastic surgeons for this type of peel is **trichloroacetic-acid, or TCA**.

The light peel is a superficial treatment that works primarily on the stratum corneum, or outer-most layer of skin. By applying the TCA solution to the properly prepared skin, the surgeon can induce the shedding of the stratum corneum, thus

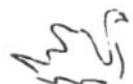

revealing the more youthful, healthier skin beneath. Don't misunderstand the term "chemical peel" - the surgeon will apply the chemical solution to your skin during your visit to his office, but the skin will not actually begin to peel for two to three days after the treatment. Just as a sunburn does not peel on the day you receive the burn, but rather a few days afterwards. Here's what you can expect to take place during the procedure:

- The first step in a light to medium chemical peel will be the cleansing of the skin. The skin surface will be first washed with soap and rinsed with water. Next, a cleanser will be used (commonly, alcohol) to degrease the skin surface. The surgeon or nurse will scrub the skin thoroughly, even spreading the folds of skin at wrinkle sites in order to degrease the body oil within the fold. (The cleansing of the skin is extremely important, since improper cleansing could cause the appearance of "frost" on the skin during the chemical application to be delayed.) This "frost", or white-ish cast to the skin color, is how the surgeon will judge the progress and/or depth of the peel.
- After all cleansing has been completed and the surgeon has prepared the skin, the doctor is ready to apply the acid solution. The surgeon will generally use a 20-35% concentration of TCA in the light peel, and may use additives. Medium peels would be done with a heavier concentration of TCA.
- The doctor will work in one area of the face (forehead, nose, etc.) at a time. The TCA solution will be applied with swabs or gauze, with the surgeon rubbing briskly along the skin surface and into the wrinkle folds.
- After a period of minutes (ranging from three to ten or so), the skin will begin to "frost" (the surface will whiten). The patient will experience a burning or stinging sensation during this period. Some surgeons will keep a small electric fan at hand, as the movement of air across the skin seems to help alleviate some of the discomfort.
- Some doctors will choose to dilute (probably with alcohol) the acid, usually within a minute or so from the onset of the frosting.
- Within a few minutes, the frosting disappears and the skin begins to redden. A deep frost can continue for up to ten or fifteen minutes, depending on the TCA concentration used, how briskly the surgeon scrubbed the skin with the solution and how many times the surgeon applied the solution. An antibiotic ointment may be applied to the treated areas. This generally helps to alleviate the discomfort.

After all areas of the face and/or body have been treated, the doctor will have you sit quietly and relax. By this point, most of the discomfort experienced

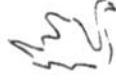

during the application of the acid has subsided, bearing in mind that you probably have been mildly sedated. With a light or medium peel, bandages are not necessary. When the surgeon feels you are up to it, you will receive some post-peel instructions and your chaffeur for the day will be allowed to take you home.

POST-TREATMENT INSTRUCTIONS - LIGHT TO MEDIUM PEEL

Before you leave the surgeon's office you will be given some important instructions to follow in the first week or so of your recovery. It is critical that these guidelines be followed closely, since improper care of the skin following a chemical peel can result in scarring or areas of abnormal pigmentation. Some of the instructions your surgeon may give you are (but be certain to follow **your** surgeon's advice):

- The face (and other treated areas) should be gently cleansed twice a day with a mild soap (your surgeon will recommend a brand) and water. **BE VERY CAREFUL - DO NOT SCRUB THE SKIN**! Use a clean container to pour warm water on the skin, then gently pat the suds that you have lathered in your hands onto the treated skin. Rinse the suds with the container of warm water. Don't stand under the shower head and allow the water to pelt the treated skin. Gently pat the area dry with a clean, soft towel. Patients can use the warm water rinse to moisten the skin as needed throughout the day.
- **Do not use moisturizers or makeup** for the period specified by your surgeon, usually from one to three days after treatment.
- The doctor will probably prescribe an antibiotic to be taken after treatment. Remember that antibiotics are generally intended to be taken until all of the prescribed capsules have been used.
- A pain medication may be prescribed, but generally is not necessary for the light to medium peels.
- Some surgeons may recommend the application of a solution to any areas of irritation that develop in the first few days after treatment. Don't take it upon yourself to treat irritation - ask your surgeon.
- The doctor may give you an ointment to be applied during the recovery period. Some do not advocate their use until two or three days following treatment, when the peeling process has gotten well underway. Remember that "gentle" is the key word in dealing with the treated areas - **never scrub, rub or pick at the treated skin during the recovery and peeling period**.
- Avoid excessive activity that may cause perspiration, try to sleep only on your back, and limit exposure to sunlight as directed by the doctor.

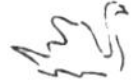

- Some itching of the treated skin may occur - **do not scratch**. Apply the prescribed ointments as directed to relieve this discomfort.
- If scabs form on the treated skin, ***do not attempt to hasten the shedding of the scab***. You risk the possibility of scarring if you "pick" at the scab!

These are generalities. The directions given to you by your surgeon should be followed closely and with care, since a substantial part of the responsibility for good healing and optimum results from your peel will depend on you. Expect feelings of tight, dry and sometimes itchy skin during the first few days.

THE PEELING AND RECOVERY PERIOD

The skin does not peel immediately after the acid is administered. Within two to three days after the chemical is applied, the treated skin will dry, crack, darken and begin to peel. It is common for the areas around the mouth and eyes to begin peeling first, since these areas are the most difficult to remain immobile during recovery (blinking, chewing and talking are difficult to avoid, no matter how hard you try). It is extremely important that the patient does not attempt to hasten the peeling process by picking or scrubbing at the peeling, flaking outer layer of skin. By indulging in this activity, the patient may expose the tender underlying skin before it is ready. This can cause localized scarring and dark, blotchy pigmentation.

Most patients who have undergone a light to medium peel are fully recovered after a week or so, sometimes within four or five days. After this period of time most of the heavy peeling has occurred, although a period of continued "flaking" may persist for a few days afterwards. Most patients can begin using makeup and their normal skin care routine after four or five days, but **check with the surgeon** to be certain. Patients should avoid unprotected exposure to the sun for a period of time recommended by their surgeon, but since sun exposure was responsible for the damage to the skin in the first place, why not continue protection as a regular routine?

Some patients will experience areas of irritation and redness, even with a light peel. The surgeon should be notified when these symptoms present themselves. Patients should try to avoid irritating the areas further. For example, if the patient has had the upper area of the chest peeled, avoiding "scratchy" materials (like some sweaters or lacy blouses) may help avoid unnecessary discomfort. To treat the irritation the surgeon will probably prescribe a soothing ointment which will relieve the condition very quickly.

Patients on a regular vitamin A derivative or glycolic acid product regimen should be able to resume their routine after a week or so following the peel, but ask your surgeon first. Indications are that patients using these products may enjoy even better results after having a peel, but be aware that use of some of these

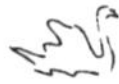

products should be avoided in irritated areas until the skin is fully healed, and only after your doctor says it's okay. Some irregularity in pigmentation has occurred in patients who applied vitamin A derivatives to skin irritated by a chemical peel.

Light peels can be repeated every few weeks, if necessary, to achieve desired results. Be aware, though, that subsequent peels should be delayed until all of the dryness, crusting and peeling from the previous peel has subsided. Reapplication of the chemical solution to skin that has not fully healed may result in a second peel that is deeper than was desired.

DEEP CHEMICAL PEELS

As we have discussed throughout this chapter, the advances made in techniques and chemical solutions have given cosmetic surgeons an opportunity to utilize a variety of peels, "customized" if you will, to the condition of the patient. For more heavily damaged skin that is exhibiting pronounced wrinkles and "lipstick lines" around the mouth, a deep chemical peel may be the best choice. Deep chemical peels can produce results that are quite dramatic: smoothing the skin, improving the complexion, and softening deep wrinkles. Of course, the deeper the peel, the greater the risk for complications and the longer the recovery period.

Currently, there are two chemicals commonly used for a deep peel. One is TCA, which we described in the Light to Medium Peel section of this chapter. To get a deeper peel with TCA the surgeon will increase the concentration of the solution, generally to 35 to 50% strength, with the highest concentrations being used on areas such as the forehead and cheeks, weaker concentrations on eyelids and neck. Indications are that TCA is one of the few chemical solutions that produce pleasing results on patients with darker skin, since it has less of a bleaching effect than phenol. In addition, TCA does not appear to be absorbed through the skin and into the system to as great a degree as phenol, reducing the potential toxicity.

The prior preparation of the skin and the application of the chemical solution in a deep TCA peel is very similar to the process used for the light or medium peel.

Precancerous lesions are generally treated with a localized deep TCA peel. In some cases, the lesion may be removed or flattened prior to the peel, in which case the surgeon will use additional care, since penetration will be greater in these pre-treated areas. Some doctors will allow a week or two for the area to heal from the lesion removal before proceeding with the peel. *Superficial* lesions can generally be treated with an acid prior to the peel, with both treatments occurring on the same day.

The other chemical commonly used by cosmetic surgeons to achieve a deep peel is **phenol**. This acid has been around for years and many surgeons still prefer

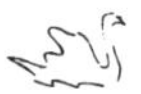

its use in deep peels, feeling that the results obtainable with phenol justify the additional care that must be taken with its use. Phenol has been proven effective on softening deep wrinkles and lines, correcting uneven pigmentation and diminishing acne scars. The best results of a phenol peel are on patients with light complexions, since it does have a distinct bleaching effect on the skin.

Because phenol is absorbed through the skin into the system, it is a potentially toxic substance. Patients with kidney or heart trouble are not viable candidates for a phenol peel. Persons who scar easily or elderly patients may also be more safely treated with another type of chemical. Patients undergoing a phenol peel should be connected to a cardiac monitor, since this substance has been known to cause heart arrythmia (uneven heart beats). Some surgeons may recommend that the patient undergo an EKG prior to treatment with phenol, to assure that no existing heart problems can be detected. ***Because of the possible side-effects of a phenol peel, patients must make absolutely certain that the substance is administered by an experienced medical professional.***

Application of the phenol will be similar to that of the TCA . At the end of the application process, however, the surgeon may elect to **tape** the treated areas. Taping allows the skin to *soak* in the solution, improving penetration and deepening the peel. Taping is much more common with a phenol peel; surgeons using TCA may not tape at all. This tape is usually removed within 48 hours after the solution is applied. Usually, tape is used only on the first peel, since subsequent peels penetrate more quickly than the initial application. Tape is seldom used on dark skinned patients. Again, the tape is generally removed within 48 hours after the chemical application.

POST-TREATMENT INSTRUCTIONS - DEEP PEELS

Patients should closely follow the guidelines given them by their plastic surgeon for the recovery period immediately following the chemical treatment. Patients who have undergone a phenol peel may be given different instructions than those that had a TCA peel. It is absolutely imperative for good healing and pleasing results that much care be taken with the affected skin.

Most of the instructions outlined for the light to medium peel apply for the deep peel, as well as some additional care:

- Ice bags placed over a clean cloth can be applied to the treated areas to alleviate swelling and discomfort. Use only in the manner approved by your surgeon.
- Steroid and/or antibiotic ointments may be prescribed to promote healing, reduce itching and limit scarring.

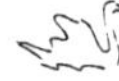

- Some patients will need a pain medication for a few days after treatment. If you need it, ask for it.
- Lubricants will probably be provided to help prevent excessive drying and cracking of the skin.
- Patients who have undergone a deep chemical peel should be prepared to avoid exposure to the sun for a minimum of three or four months. Your skin will be extremely sensitive during this period, and protection is absolutely necessary. Uneven pigmentation can occur as a result of sun exposure.

Again, these are generalities - your post-operative instructions will differ if you have had a phenol peel. The directions given you by your cosmetic surgeon should be followed closely and with care, since a large part of the responsibility for good healing and optimum results from your peel falls on you. Expect to be somewhat uncomfortable initially, and to not look your best for least a week or so.

THE PEELING AND RECOVERY PERIOD

As with the lighter peels, the skin will go through a "damaged" phase prior to beginning to peel. The process is longer with the deeper peel, and the effects of the acid burn are much more pronounced.

When the tape (if the surgeon used it) is removed (usually within 48 hours after treatment) the skin will be very pink and swollen, with a moist appearance. Early removal of the tape is not advisable since it can be extremely uncomfortable for the patient and can cause localized bleeding. After the tape is removed, a varying degree of scabbing and crusting of the treated skin will be experienced, followed by a period of redness and swelling as the scab comes off.

With the deep TCA peel, the redness and swelling should diminish in seven to fourteen days, but the skin may continue to flake for a period of several weeks, especially treated skin on the chest or arms. The surgeon will probably prescribe ointments to help prevent excessive drying and cracking of the healing skin.

Patients who have received a **phenol** peel usually experience heavier scabbing after the surgical tape is removed from the treated areas. In fact, don't be surprised if a thick scab forms over the entire treated area. Within a week, the scab will shed (**do not attempt to facilitate the shedding of the scab by "picking" or scratching!**) and the skin will have a bright red, swollen appearance. The swelling from the phenol peel generally takes between three and six weeks to fully subside, and the redness can diminish gradually over a period of up to a couple of months.

Once the swelling and redness disappear, the skin is usually much smoother and tighter than before the peel. Patience is required in healing from a deep

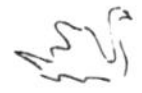

chemical peel, and the patient must be prepared for a recovery period that is lengthier than that experienced with a light peel.

RISKS AND COMPLICATIONS

As with most medical treatments, there are risks and complications to be considered when undergoing a chemical peel. Certain chemicals carry more risks than others, but patients must remember that a very potent substance is going to be applied to their skin in order to create a controlled burn of the outer layer(s) of skin. Patients must be extremely cautious in selecting the person who will administer this acid - a licensed, board certified, *experienced* medical professional specializing in these types of treatments is the *only* type of surgeon that you should consider in your selection process. Even in lighter concentrations, these chemicals, if improperly applied or monitored, can induce permanent scarring.

Be certain to ask your cosmetic surgeon how many peels he or she has done with this substance and in this concentration. Ask to see "before and after" pictures of patients who have undergone similar treatment with similar solutions. Since many of these techniques are somewhat new, experience should be very important in your selection process.

Some of the risks and complications that should be considered in undergoing a chemical peel are:

- **Uneven pigmentation** is most commonly seen in persons with darker skin. These will appear as blotchy areas, and are sometimes due to uneven penetration of the acid or an incident which occurred in the healing process. Some localized abnormal pigmentation can be corrected with subsequent treatment.
- **Scarring,** either due to excessive penetration of the acid, or through improper care during the peel and healing process, is possible. These scars may be permanent and difficult to treat.
- **Sun Sensitivity** is to be expected, especially in the deeper peels. Some patients who have undergone phenol peels may be extremely sensitive for an extended period of time.
- **Unnatural skin appearance**, namely a "waxy" look to the complexion, occurs in some patients who have undergone a deep peel.
- **Bleaching of the Skin** does occur with phenol peels. On patients with darker complexions, this can create a marked difference in skin color between the treated and untreated areas. The face, for example, will be considerably lighter in color than the neck, chest and arms. Some patients will find it necessary to use makeup to compensate for the difference in skin color on a permanent, ongoing basis.

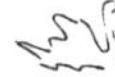

- **Skin Sensitivity** occurs in some patients, in that the treated areas can become irritated more easily after the chemical peel. Some patients experience an increased sensitivity to the changes in pigmentation that some drugs can induce, such as estrogen, birth control pills and the antibiotic, tetracycline.
- **Infection** is a possibility, although a rare occurrence, provided the patient takes care to take all of the antibiotics prescribed by the doctor and exercises proper care during the recovery process.
- **Toxicity** is primarily a problem with phenol peels, since TCA is thought to be not as readily or as easily absorbed through the skin and into the system. Patients have experienced irregular heartbeats during the application of phenol. Persons with heart or kidney problems should not consider phenol a viable option.
- **Vision damage** has occurred in some chemical peels, although very rarely. In such cases, the solution has penetrated through the eyelid and onto the cornea.

These are some of the risks and complications that should be considered when undergoing a chemical peel. The list is by no means complete, and you are encouraged to discuss possible risks in detail with your cosmetic surgeon prior to consenting to the procedure.

COST OF CHEMICAL PEELS

Because of the variety of chemical peels now in use by cosmetic surgeons, there is a wide range of fees being charged for this type of treatment. According to the American Society of Plastic and Reconstructive Surgeons, the **average** surgeon's fees reported by members for a full face chemical peel performed in 1990 was **$1640.** However, bear in mind that charges on the east and west coasts are generally higher, with the least expensive procedures available in the interior regions of the U.S. These are generalities and should not be used to measure the fees charged by your surgeon.

The vast majority of chemical peels are done on an outpatient basis, under mild or heavy sedation rather than general anesthesia. This helps keep the cost down on the procedure, since a hospital stay is generally not necessary.

In addition, a series of light peels may be the recommended treatment for your skin. If this is true in your case, the fees may be slightly higher or lower, depending on the number of peels the physician feels will be necessary. ***Make certain the fees quoted to you* include *any pre-peel skin preparations and follow-up treatment*.** The cost of prescription drugs needed for the preparation period may

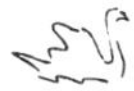

not be included, of course, as well as any post-peel skin care products recommended for your use by the cosmetic surgeon.

As with all cosmetic surgery procedures, make certain that you understand the total cost of the chemical peel prior to agreeing to treatment. Most insurance companies **do not** cover surgery or treatment undertaken for purely cosmetic reasons. If you are having a chemical peel to remove precancerous lesions, however, talk to your surgeon and your insurance company prior to treatment. This type of procedure *may* be covered.

ANESTHESIA

Most chemical peels, ranging from the lightest to deepest treatments, are done under sedation only. Phenol peels, as a rule, are more painful and will require heavier sedation. Some plastic surgeons will provide the patient with a tranquilizer to be taken prior to coming to the office for the peel. Immediately prior to the peel, an injection of a narcotic may be given to calm the nerves and relax the patient. When the light TCA solutions are to be administered, no sedation may be necessary.

Very few patients require heavier sedation than that described above. It is not unheard of, however, for an intravenous sedation to be administered to patients who are extremely nervous about the procedure or complain of severe discomfort during the application of the chemical solution. Discuss with your cosmetic surgeon what types of sedation and pain medication will be used both before and during the procedure.

Some surgeons will prescribe a pain medication to be taken on an "as needed" basis for a couple of days after the procedure. This is definitely more common when the patient has undergone a deep peel, such as one done with phenol.

POST-PEEL SKIN CARE

As we mentioned earlier in the chapter, indications are that the effects of vitamin A derivatives, glycolic acid products and other deep penetrating skin care products are increased after the patient has undergone a chemical peel. With the removal of the thickened ***stratum corneum*** (outer layer of skin), the penetration of the products into the skin is greatly enhanced, just as the use of these products in the preparation process prior to the chemical peel greatly enhances the penetration of the peel solution.

A number of plastic surgeons are using vitamin A products and alpha-hydroxy acid (lactic acid and glycolic acid) products as part of a complete skin program, designed to prepare the skin for the peel, undo the damage that currently exists and to maintain the smoother, younger-looking skin achieved by the peel.

Some of the key steps in a total-care program recommended by some doctors are:

1. Begin preparing the skin for the peel process by using vitamin A products or products containing glycolic acid.
2. Perform a light, medium or deep peel, depending on the condition of the skin. The lighter TCA peels can be repeated as necessary to achieve the desired results.
3. After all irritation from the peel has subsided, the patient resumes the use of vitamin A and/or glycolic acid products, constantly shedding the dead cells of the stratum corneum and preventing the thickening process of this outer layer of skin that contributes to the dry, scaly, ruddy appearance of the complexion. In addition, some medical professionals, along with the manufacturers of the glycolic acid products, indicate that these products may help regenerate collagen and elastin in the skin.
4. Patients must maintain a program that protects the skin from sun damage. Most cosmetic surgeons recommend at least a SPF 15 level product, to be used on a daily basis.

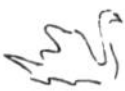

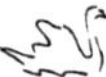

CHAPTER TWELVE

NON-SURGICAL TECHNIQUES FOR YOUNGER-LOOKING SKIN

"Fine Art is that in which the hand, the head and the heart of man go together."

John Ruskin
The Two Paths (1859),2.

According to data gathered by the American Society of Plastic and Reconstructive Surgeons from its members, about half of all cosmetic surgery performed in the United States is undertaken by patients that are striving to improve the appearance of an aging face. As we discussed in Chapter Eleven, the factors most to blame for the visible signs of aging are **sun damage and gravity**. To better understand how skin ages, you should review the first few pages of Chapter Eleven.

Gravity can take credit for the sagging and drooping of skin, while the effects of sun damage are manifested by fine lines and wrinkles, a sallow tone to the complexion, uneven pigmentation, and a rough appearance to the skin. The effects of sun damage are those that present themselves first, and respond best to non-surgical treatments.

There are a number of products and techniques currently being used in an effort to reverse some of the signs of photo-aging (caused by sun exposure). They range from a simple daily routine of cleansing, moisturizing and sunscreen protection up to the more drastic repair measures, such as a chemical peel.

Skin care professionals, including cosmetic surgeons and dermatologists, are now beginning to stress the importance of a holistic approach to maintaining beautiful skin and therefore a more youthful, healthy appearance. ***Prevention, correction*** and ***maintenance*** are the keys to younger looking skin.

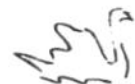

PREVENTION

As the old saying goes, "an ounce of prevention is worth a pound of cure". Scientists are finding that even sun damage experienced very early in life, in the childhood years, has an effect on the condition of adult skin, and may predispose certain people to skin cancers. It cannot be stressed enough that protection from the harmful rays of the sun must be a daily practice, and must begin early in life. Teenagers seen baking in the sun today will pay the price tomorrow, with aging, leathery skin and a possible threat to their good health.

Since the damaging effects of the sun are usually the first visible signs of an aging face, it is logical to say that by preventing the damage we can greatly delay the appearance of fine lines and wrinkles and therefore maintain a more youthful appearance for a longer period of time. Protecting the skin from sun damage is a full time job - experts say that the majority of cellular damage comes from every day exposure, not those weekends that you don a bikini and bake in the sun, as you may think.

For everyday use most skin care experts recommend a sunscreen with an SPF ranging from 6 to 15. Higher SPF levels can irritate sensitive skin when used on a daily basis, so find a product in the recommended range that is comfortable for you and **use it daily**. While sunbathing, most people should use a full-spectrum sunscreen containing at least an SPF 30 in order to fully protect against both sunburn and *cellular damage*. Full-spectrum products effectively prevent penetration of both Ultraviolet A and Ultraviolet B rays (UV-A damages collagen and elastin deep in the skin, UV-B causes sunburns).

By preventing further sun damage you can slow the clock on aging. If you are already beginning to show signs of photo-aging, there are options open to you that can help reduce the visible evidence of your lack of prior skin protection.

CORRECTION OF EXISTING DAMAGE

It sometimes seems as though there is a "new and improved" method of fighting aging skin with the rising of every full moon. Some products and procedures are legitimate and truly result in improvement, while others are merely repackaged moisturizers or vitamin creams.

We fully encourage every reader to visit a medical professional (preferably a dermatologist or plastic surgeon) for a full evaluation of what is needed and safe for use in their unique circumstances before using any of these products or procedures. Self-treatment can be hazardous to your good looks and your health.

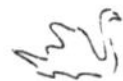

GLYCOLIC ACID

A large number of skin care professionals feel that one of the most promising developments in helping to reverse and prevent the signs of aging due to sun damage is the use of products containing *Alphahydroxy acids*. So far, the most popular of these naturally-occurring acids that are present in such substances as milk and apples is ***glycolic acid***, found in sugar cane.

A number of reliable sources ranging from dermatological publications to skin care professionals are expressing confidence and excitement about the use of products containing glycolic acid in the fight against fine lines and wrinkles, "age" spots, skin discolorations and even mild scars. By breaking down some of the adhesive properties of the outer layer of skin, glycolic acid promotes the shedding of the dead cells in the stratum corneum. The skin takes on a smoother, healthier appearance and may have the glowing radiance that usually is present in a much younger face.

So far, glycolic acid appears to have a broader appeal to a greater number of people than does some prescription products. It appears to be much less irritating so that even patients with sensitive skin can use the products. It penetrates more easily into the skin due to a smaller molecular structure, so it can be more effective. It is not a prescription drug, and the cost of daily use can be much less expensive. Fewer patients experience heavy flaking of the skin with glycolic acid, and it is reported to not make the skin as sun-sensitive as some prescription drugs. Plan on using these products for around three months before seeing substantially noticeable results.

There are two companies currently licensed to market glycolic acid products in the formulations which appear to be the most effective in reducing the signs of aging. **M.D. Formulations™** a line developed by Herald Pharmaceutical, were the first to actively promote a skin care product containing glycolic acid. M.D. *Formulations*™ distributes only through skin care professionals such as dermatologists, cosmetic surgeons and salons. They have a wide range of products containing glycolic acid that range in retail price from $25 for a facial cleanser to $60 for a night cream. Most people would use the cleanser in the morning followed by the Facial Lotion, and again at night before applying the Night Cream. The facial lotion is of thinner texture, while the Night Cream is of a richer consistency.

The younger of the two companies marketing glycolic acid products is **NeoStrata®**. Formed as a result of years of research on the part on a prominent physician and a scientist who experienced consistently positive results, *NeoStrata*® is a progressive company that appears to be dedicated to increasing awareness about the benefits of glycolic acid products. Acknowledging that we, the consumer,

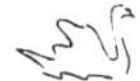

are constantly bombarded with "miracle cures" for aging, *NeoStrata*® has taken a conservative approach in promoting their products in the recent past - they primarily targeted dermatologists and other medical professionals, slowly building confidence and expertise within the medical community and fine-tuning their product line. The focus of *NeoStrata*®'s distribution process is through dermatologists and other medical professionals, but they plan to begin offering their products in drug stores in mid-1992, recognizing that consumer demand will increase as awareness of their products becomes more wide-spread.

NeoStrata® offers a product line that varies in concentration and consistency. The cornerstone of their line is the **AHA** (Alphahydroxy acid) **Skin Smoothing Lotion**, a translucent lotion of substantial concentration that is used twice daily. Other products include the **AHA Enhanced Gel Formula** which provides relief for the dry, rough and thickened skin on the hands and feet; **AHA Gel** for Age Spots and Skin Lightening - works effectively on age or "liver" spots, freckles and areas of uneven pigmentation such as the "mask of pregnancy". An acne solution and Skin Smoothing Cream is also available.

COLLAGEN INJECTIONS

After years of wear, tear and sun damage, the skin begins to lose its underlying support system, made up of primarily collagen and elastin. As a result of this loss of support the skin will collapse, and ***ta-da!*** - a wrinkle is born. In the past few years, plastic surgeons and dermatologists have seen a dramatic increase in the consumer demand for collagen replacement. In the ten or so years since the FDA approved its use in 1981, over a half million people have had collagen injection treatments. In fact, it is now the most popular of the anti-aging non-surgical procedures, according to the 1990 figures reported to the American Society of Plastic and Reconstructive Surgeons by its members. Over 80,000 collagen injection procedures were performed in that year by members of the ASPRS.

The collagen used in these types of procedures is actually derived from cow skin. It's content is mostly water, but the substance is reportedly very close in composition to that of human collagen and is more likely accepted by the body. A couple of different types of collagen are currently in use. The type used in your treatment will depend on the area of the face to be treated and the depth of the depression (wrinkle or scar).

A number of patients experience an allergic reaction to the substance, however, and are not viable candidates for the injection procedure. All patients should have an allergy test prior to the procedure, and some experts recommend **two** pre-treatment skin tests. Most physicians will do one on the day of your consultation. Be certain to monitor the test area thoroughly for the four-week test

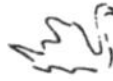

period. By not reporting a reaction to your doctor, you could be letting yourself in for a more severe allergic reaction after treatment.

Once a skin test has been completed with no reactions, the doctor will begin your treatments. Since collagen treatments are not permanent in most cases, the normal patient will require a treatment every few months or so in order to maintain the desired results.

During the procedure, the doctor will inject a small amount of collagen under the skin into the area of the depression (acne scar, wrinkle, etc.). The injected substance will act with the body's own collagen to plump up the wrinkle, bringing the skin over the injected area up to the desired level.

Virtually all collagen injection procedures are done on an outpatient basis, with an average fee range of about $250 to $600 per treatment. Most patients will need more than one treatment to achieve the desired results.

Be certain to discuss the risks and possible complications of collagen injection with your dermatologist or cosmetic surgeon. While most complications (other than allergic reaction) are fairly rare, there have been a few cases of infection, bruising and/or scarring, blockage of blood flow and subsequent tissue damage, visibility of the injected material (white and/or raised bump), nausea, rash, headache, difficulty in breathing or joint pain. Again, most of these are extremely rare - but discuss all risks and complications with your doctor before consenting to treatment.

FAT AND OTHER INJECTIBLES

For a period, the injection of other materials, such as a person's own fat tissue or silicone, were almost entirely replaced by the use of collagen. While there is very little risk of allergic reaction in using fat, the medical community seemed to agree that the results are of such a temporary nature that it almost wasn't worth the trouble or expense of treatment. About 8,000 or so patients underwent fat injection procedures in 1990, according to the members of the ASPRS. Even though collagen injections are temporary, too, some fat injection patients have results that last scarcely a couple of months before the injections must be repeated. There is continued research in using a patient's own tissue for wrinkle repair, however, so you can anticipate more progress in that department, and may see injection of a patient's own fat into wrinkles and fine lines regain some popularity.

Silicone injection has all but gone the way of the dinosaur, with surgeons abandoning this substance due the problems experienced in the past; some patients ended up with permanent raised bumps from the injections and other serious complications. The newest silicone scare, with some medical professionals of the opinion that the silicone can move through the body and cause damage or affect the autoimmune system, has all but eliminated it's use for this type of procedure. Most experts feel that silicone injection is not a viable alternative for human injection.

MAINTENANCE

Most of the keys to maintaining beautiful, healthy-looking skin are the things that your skin would tell you if it could talk:

- Moisturize when your skin feels dry and taut. It won't hurt to use a moisturizer every day, since they tend to "plump up" the skin cells.
- Exfoliate on a regular basis to help shed the old cells of the outer most layers. Some skin care professionals feel that a damp wash cloth is all the abrasion that is needed.
- Continue using protection from the sun. This alone will help keep a more youthful appearance to the skin.
- Use a mild soap and rinse your skin thoroughly; remove all make-up before retiring for the night.
- Stop smoking and limit alcohol consumption - these two factors can age you beyond your years *in a hurry*.
- Maintain a healthy diet and regular exercise program. Your skin has a way of reflecting your overall health, so taking care of yourself is the best way to keep your skin looking it's best!

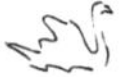

GLOSSARY

abdominoplasty - or tummy tuck, is surgery performed to correct a sagging abdomen by the removal of excess skin and fat, and sometimes the drawing together of muscles (Chapter 9).

blepharoplasty - the eyelid procedure (Chapter 3).

breast augmentation - a procedure whereby the breast is augmented, or added to, with an implant device. Also called breast enlargement (Chapter 7).

breast reduction - the procedure used to reduce the size of the breasts by removal of fat, skin and breast tissue (Chapter 6).

breast uplift - (also called mastopexy) the procedure in which skin is removed from the breast and the nipple repositioned in order to correct a sagging, pendulous appearance. Some surgeons refer to this as the ptosis procedure - ptosis meaning "droop" or "sag" (Chapter 8).

chin augmentation - the procedure in which an implant device is placed within the chin to enhance projection of that facial area (Chapter 5).

collagen - found throughout our bodies, collagen is a strong, fibrous protein which performs structural and connective functions. Loss of collagen in skin tissue can contribute to wrinkles and fine lines (Chapter 11 and 12).

dermatologist - a doctor specializing in treating the skin, and who may be experienced in performing chemical peels and other non-surgical techniques.

dermis - *or corium*: the inner layers of the skin which contain blood vessels, nerves, sweat and subaceous (oil) glands.

epidermis - the outer layers of the skin which are made up of four sub-layers, ranging from the outermost to the innermost:

- the stratum cornuem (see definition)
- the "clean" layer
- the granular layer
- the malpighian layer

elastin - a strong protein found in the fibers of connective tissue throughout the body.

liposuction - the surgical removal of localized fat deposits utilizing suction mechanisms (Chapter 10).

mastopexy - the breast uplift procedure (Chapter 8).

ophthalmologist - eye specialist who may be trained in cosmetic eyelid surgery.

otolaryngologist - an eye, nose and throuat doctor who may be trained in performing cosmetic procedures on the nose and ears.

reduction mammoplasty - the breast reduction procedure (Chapter 6).

rhinoplasty - the nose reshaping procedure (chapter 5).

rhytidectomy - the facelift procedure (Chapter 4).

silicone implants - a number of different types of devices that commonly include a rubber-silicone outer shell filled with silicone gel. These devices are used in such procedures as breast enlargement and reconstruction (Chapter 7).

skin - made up of two main parts: the epidermis, or outermost layers, and the corium, or dermis, the innermost layers.

stratum corneum - the outermost layer of the epidermis, made up of dead skin cells which are constantly shedding and being replaced by new cells from deeper within the epidermis.

suction lipectomy - see liposuction above (Chapter 10).

trichloroacetic acid - *or* TCA, is a substance currently being used to perform chemical peels on the skin in order to reduce the effects of sun damage (Chapter 11).

tummy tuck - see abdominoplasty above (Chapter 9).

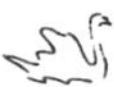

INDEX

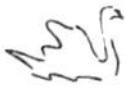

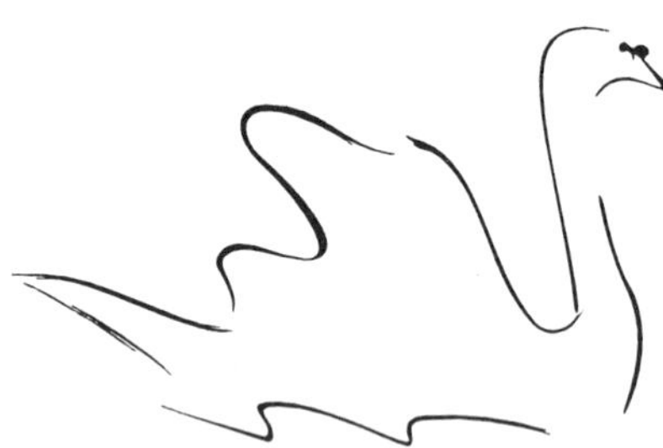

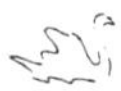

Order Form

Please send me ☐ copies of

Cosmetic Surgery:
The Consumer's Complete Easy Guide from Before to After

Name: ______________________________

Address: ______________________________

____

City: ______________________________

State: ____________ **ZIP Code:** ____________

Florida Addresses: Please enclose 6% state sales tax

Enclosed is a check or money order for $16.95 plus $1.95 shipping and handling for each book.

Mail Order Form and Check or Money Order to:

Swan Park Publishing
Post Office Box 574496
Orlando, FL 32857-4496

Please allow 4 – 6 weeks for shipping

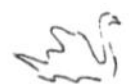